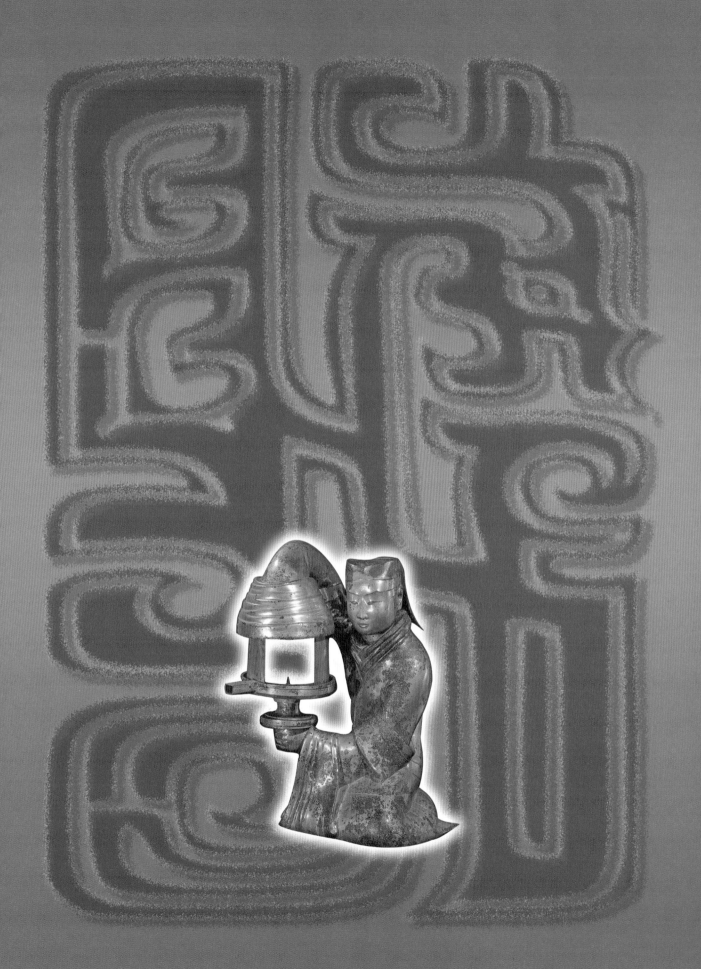

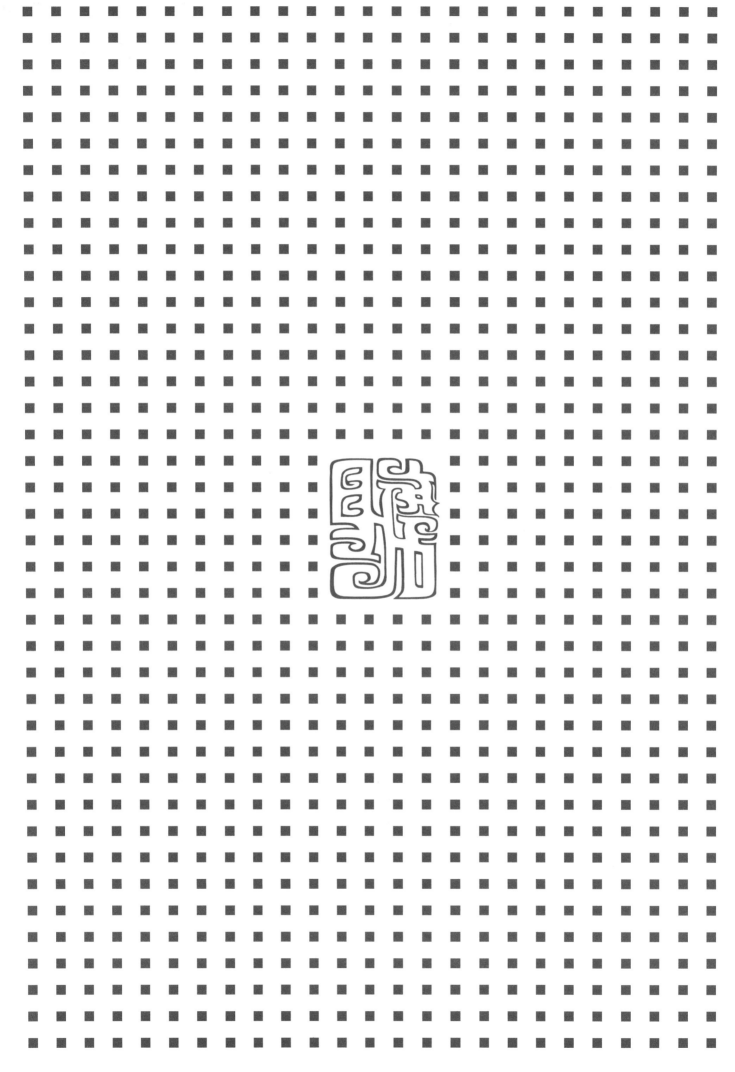

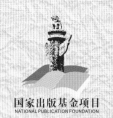

国家出版基金项目
NATIONAL PUBLICATION FOUNDATION

中华医药卫生

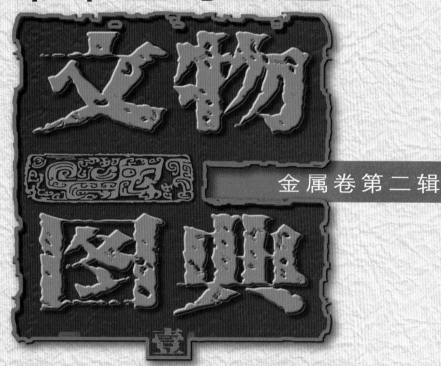

金属卷第二辑

主　编　李经纬　梁　峻　刘学春
总主译　白永权
主　译　聂文信

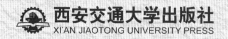

西安交通大学出版社
XI'AN JIAOTONG UNIVERSITY PRESS

图书在版编目（CIP）数据

中华医药卫生文物图典 . 1. 金属卷 . 第 2 辑 . / 李经纬、
梁峻，刘学春主编 . — 西安：西安交通大学出版社，2016.12

ISBN 978-7-5605-7024-2

Ⅰ . ①中… Ⅱ . ①李… ②梁… ③刘… Ⅲ . ①中国医药学—
金属器物—古器物—中国—图录 Ⅳ . ① R-092 ② K870.2

中国版本图书馆 CIP 数据核字（2015）第 022422 号

书　　名　中华医药卫生文物图典（一）金属卷第二辑
主　　编　李经纬　梁　峻　刘学春
责任编辑　李　晶

出版发行　西安交通大学出版社
　　　　　（西安市兴庆南路 10 号　邮政编码 710049）
网　　址　http://www.xjtupress.com
电　　话　（029）82668805　82668502（医学分社）
　　　　　（029）82668315（总编办）
传　　真　（029）82668280
印　　刷　中煤地西安地图制印有限公司

开　　本　889mm×1194mm　1/16　印张 29.5　字数　462 千字
版次印次　2017 年 12 月第 1 版　2017 年 12 月第 1 次印刷
书　　号　ISBN 978-7-5605-7024-2
定　　价　880.00 元

读者购书、书店添货、如发现印装质量问题，请通过以下方式联系、调换。

订购热线：（029）82665248　（029）82665249
投稿热线：（029）82668805　（029）82668502
读者信箱：medpress@126.com

铭记感受历史

自信自重自强自强

中华医药卫生文物图典问世

书贺

陈可冀谨题

二〇一七年春月

陈可冀　中国科学院院士、国医大师

精修醫藥衛生文物

圖典功著當代

深究岐黃學術思想

淵源惠澤千秋

中華醫藥衛生文物圖典出版誌慶

丁酉孟秋 孫光榮 敬題於北京

孙光荣　国医大师

中華醫藥衛生文物圖典出版

彰顯中醫藥
文化精神

體現中醫藥
歷史价值

歲次丁酉夏 王琦

王琦　国医大师

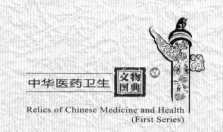

中华医药卫生文物图典（一）
丛书编撰委员会

主　编　李经纬　梁　峻　刘学春

副主编　廖　果　吴鸿洲　康兴军　和中浚　刘小斌　杨金生

　　　　　郑怀林　徐江雁　白建疆　黄　煌

编　委　李洪晓　梁永宣　王强虎　董树平　马　健　王　霞

　　　　　张雅宗　朱德明　包哈申　张建青　郑　蓉　庄乾竹

　　　　　李宏红　刘哲峰　王宏才　陈润东

总主译　白永权

主　译　陈向京　聂文信　范晓晖　温　睿　赵永生　杜彦龙

　　　　　吉　乐　李小棉　郭　梦　陈　曦

副主译（按姓氏音序排列）

　　　　　董艳云　姜雨孜　李建西　刘　慧　马　健　任宝磊

　　　　　任　萌　任　莹　王　颇　习通源　谢皖吉　徐素云

　　　　　许崇钰　许　梅　詹菊红　赵　菲　邹郝晶

译 者（按姓氏音序排列）

迟征宇　邓　甜　付一豪　高　琛　高　媛　郭　宁

韩　蕾　何宗昌　胡勇强　黄　鋆　蒋新蕾　康晓薇

李静波　刘雅恬　刘妍萌　鲁显生　马　月　牛笑语

唐云鹏　唐臻娜　田　多　铁红玲　佟健一　王　晨

王　丹　王　栋　王　丽　王　媛　王慧敏　王梦杰

王仙先　吴耀均　席　慧　肖国强　许子洋　闫红贤

杨姣姣　姚　晔　张　阳　张　鋆　张继飞　张梦原

张晓谦　赵　欣　赵亚力　郑　青　郑艳华　朱江嵩

朱瑛培

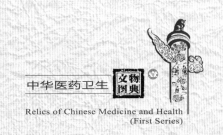

中华医药卫生 文物图典

Relics of Chinese Medicine and Health
(First Series)

本册编撰委员会

主　编　李经纬　梁　峻　刘学春

副主编　廖　果　吴鸿洲　康兴军　和中浚　刘小斌　杨金生
　　　　　郑怀林　徐江雁　白建疆　黄　煌

编　委　李洪晓　梁永宣　王强虎　董树平　马　健　王　霞
　　　　　张雅宗　朱德明　包哈申　张建青　郑　蓉　庄乾竹
　　　　　李宏红　刘哲峰　王宏才　陈润东

总主译　白永权

主　译　聂文信

副主译　姜雨孜

译　者　唐臻娜　王慧敏　迟征宇　张梦原　高　琛　王　媛
　　　　　牛笑语　吴耀均　黄　銎　杨姣姣　蒋新蕾　席　慧

丛书策划委员会

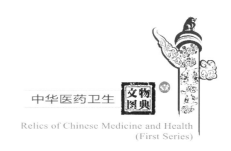

中华医药卫生 文物图典

Relics of Chinese Medicine and Health
(First Series)

序　言

　　探索天、地、人运动变化规律以及"气化物生"过程的相互关系，是人类永恒的课题。宇宙不可逆，地球不可逆，人生不可逆业已成为共识。天地造化形成自然，人类活动构成文化。文物既是文化的载体，又是物化的历史，还是文明的见证。

　　追求健康长寿是人类共同的夙愿。中华民族之所以繁衍昌盛，健康文化起了巨大的推动作用。由于古人谋求生存发展、应对环境变化产生的智慧，大多反映在以医药卫生为核心的健康文化之中，所以，习总书记说："中医药学是中国古代科学的瑰宝，也是打开中华文明宝库的钥匙"。

　　秉持文化大发展、大繁荣理念，中国中医科学院李经纬、梁峻等为负责人的科研团队在完成科技部"国家重点医药卫生文物收集调研和保护"课题获 2005 年度中华中医药学会科技二等奖基础上，又资鉴"夏商周断代工程""中华文明探源工程"等相关考古成果，用有重要价值的新出土文物置换原拍摄质量较差的文物，适当补充民族医药文物，共精选收载 5000 余件。经西安交通大学出版社申报，《中华医药卫生文物图典（一）》（以下简称《图典》）于 2013 年获得了国家出版基金的资助，并经专业翻译团队翻译，使《图典》得以面世。

　　文物承载的信息多元丰富，发掘解读其中蕴藏的智慧并非易事。医药卫生文物更具有特殊性，除文物的一般属性外，还承载着传统医学发展史迹与促进健康的信息。运用历史唯物主义观察发掘文物信息，善于从生活文物中领悟卫生信息，才能准确解读其功能，也才能诠释其在民生健康中的历史作用，收到以古鉴今之效果。"历史是现实的根源"，任何一个民族都不能割断历史，史料都包含在文化中。"文化是民族的血脉，是人民的精神家园"，文化繁荣才能实现中华民族的伟大复兴。值本《图典》付梓之际，用"梳理文化之脉，必获健康之果"作为序言并和作者、读者共勉！

中央文史研究馆馆员
中国工程院院士　　王永炎
丁酉年仲夏

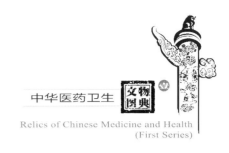

中华医药卫生文物图典

Relics of Chinese Medicine and Health
(First Series)

前　言

　　文化是相对自然的概念，是考古界常用词汇。文物是文化的重要组成部分，既是文明的物证，又是物化的历史。狭义医药卫生文物是疾病防治模式语境下的解读，而广义医药卫生文物则是躯体、心态、环境适应三维健康模式下的诠释。中华民族是56个民族组成的多元一体大家庭，中华医药卫生文物当然包括各民族的健康文化遗存。

　　天地造化如造山、板块漂移、气候变迁、生物起源进化等形成自然。气化物生莫贵于人，即整个生物进化的最高成果是人类自身。广义而言，人类生存思维留下的痕迹即物质财富和精神财富总和构成文化，其一般的物化形式是视觉感知的文物、文献、胜迹等。其中质变标志明晰的文化如文字、文物、城市、礼仪等可称作文明。从唯物史观视角观察，狭义文化即精神财富，尤其体现人类精、气、神状态的事项，其本质也具有特殊物质属性，如量子也具有波粒二相性，这种粒子也是物质，无非运动方式特殊而已。现代所谓可重复验证的"科学"，事实上也是从文化中分离出来的事项，因此也是一种特殊文化形式。追求健康长寿是人类共同的夙愿。中华民族之所以繁衍昌盛，是因为健康文化异彩纷呈。中华优秀传统医药文化之所以博大精深，是因为其原创思维博大、格物致知精深，所以，习总书记说："中医药学是中国古代科学的瑰宝，也是打开中华文明宝库的钥匙"。

文化既反映时代、地域、民族分布、生产资料来源、技术水平等信息，又反映人类认知水平和生存智慧。发掘解读文物、文献中蕴藏的健康知识和灵动智慧，首先是从事健康工作者的责任和义务。《易经》设有"观"卦，人类作为观察者，不仅要积极收藏展陈文物，而且要善于捕捉文物倾诉的信息，汲取养分，启迪思维，收到古为今用之效果。墨子三表法，首先一表即"本之于古者圣王之事"，也是强调古代史实的重要性。"历史是现实的根源"，现实是未来的基础。任何一个国家、地区、民族都不能割断历史、忽略基础，这个基础就是文化。"文化是民族的血脉，是人民的精神家园"。文化繁荣才能驱动各项事业发展，才能实现中华民族的伟大复兴。

人类从类人猿分化出来。"禄丰古猿禄丰种"是云南禄丰发现的类人猿化石，距今七八百万年。距今 200 万年前人类进入旧石器时代，直立行走，打制石器产生工具意识，管理火种，是所谓"燧人氏"时代。中国留存有更新世早、中期的元谋、蓝田、北京人等遗址。距今 10 万—5 万年前，人类进入旧石器时代中期，即早期智人阶段，脑容量增加，和欧洲、非洲人种相比，原始蒙古人种颧骨前突等，是所谓"伏羲氏"时代。中国发现的马坝、长阳、丁村人等较典型。距今 5 万—1 万年前，人类进入旧石器时代晚期，即晚期智人阶段，细石器、骨角器等遍布全国，山顶洞、柳江、资阳人等较典型。

中石器时代距今约 1 万年，是旧石器时代向新石器时代的短暂过渡期，弓箭发明，狗被驯化。河南灵井、陕西沙苑遗址等作为代表。距今 1 万—公元前 2600 年前后，人类进入新石器时代，磨光石器、烧制陶器，出现农业村落并饲养家畜，是所谓"神农氏"时代。公元前 7000 年以来，在甲、骨、陶、石等载体上出现契刻符号、七音阶骨笛乐器等，反映出人文气息趋浓。公元前 6000—公元前 3500 年的老官台、裴李岗、河姆渡、马家浜、仰韶等文化遗址，彰显出先民围绕生存健康问题所做的各种努力。

公元前 4800 年以来，以关中、晋南、豫西为中心形成的仰韶文化，是中原史前文化的重要标志。以半坡、庙底沟类型为典型，自公元前 3500 年走向繁荣，属于锄耕粟黍稻兼营渔猎饲养猪鸡经济方式，彩陶尤其发达。公元前 4400—公元前 3300 年，长江中游的大溪文化，薄胎彩陶和白陶发达。公元前 4300—公元前 2500 年山东丰岛的大汶口文化，红陶为主。公元前 3500 年前后，辽东的红山文化原始宗教发展。公元前 3300 年以来，长江下游由河姆渡、马家浜文化衍续的良渚文化和陇西的马家窑文化、江淮间的薛家岗文化时趋发达。

公元前 2600—公元前 2000 年，黄河中下游龙山文化群形成，冶铸铜器，制作玉器，土坯、石灰、夯筑技术开始应用。公元前 2697 年，轩辕战败炎帝（有说其后裔）、蚩尤而为黄帝纪元元年。黄帝西巡访贤，"至岐见岐伯，引载而归，访于治道"。其引归地"溱洧襟带于前，梅泰环拱于后"，即今河南新密市古城寨。岐黄答问，构建《黄帝内经》健康知识体系，中华文明从关注民生健康起步。颛顼改革宗教，神职人员出现；帝喾修身节用，帝尧和合百国，舜同律度量衡，大禹疏导治水，中华民族不断繁衍昌盛。

公元前 2070 年，禹之子启以豫西晋南为中心建立夏王朝，二里头青铜文化为其特征，半地穴、窑洞、地面建筑并存。饮食卫生器具、酒器增多。朱砂安神作用在宫殿应用。公元前 1600 年，商灭夏。偃师商城设有铸铜作坊。公元前 1300 年，盘庚迁殷，使用甲骨文。武丁时期青铜浑铸、分铸并存。公元前 1056 年，相传周"文王被殷纣拘于羑里，演《周易》，成六十四卦"。公元前 1046 年，武王克商建周，定都镐京。青铜器始铸长篇铭文，周原发掘出微型甲骨文字。公元前 770 年，平王东迁。虢国铸铜柄铁剑。公元前 753 年，秦国设置史官。公元前 707 年出现蝗灾、公元前 613 年出现"哈雷彗星"，均被孔子载入《春秋》。公元前 221 年，秦始皇统一中国，多元一体民族大家庭形成，中华医药卫生文物异彩纷呈。

中国是治史大国，历来重视发展文化博物事业，1955 年成立卫生部中医研究院时就设置医史研究室，1982 年中国医史文献研究所成立时复建中国医史博物馆研究收藏展陈文物。2000—2003 年，经王永炎院士、姚乃礼院长等呼吁，科技部批准立项，由李经纬、梁峻为负责人的团队完成"国家重点医药卫生文物收集调研和保护"项目任务，受到科技部项目验收组专家的高度评价，获中华中医药学会科技进步二等奖。2013 年，在国家出版基金资助下，课题组对部分文物重新拍摄或必要置换、充实民族医药文物后，由西安交通大学出版社编辑、组聘国内一流翻译团队英译说明文字付梓，受到国家中医药博物馆筹备工作领导小组和办公室的高度重视。

"物以类聚"，《图典》主要依据文物质地、种类分为 9 卷，计有陶瓷，金属，纸质，竹木，玉石、织品及标本，壁画石刻及遗址，少数民族文物，其他，备考等卷。同卷下主要根据历史年代或小类分册设章。每卷下的历史时段不求统一。遵循上述规则将《图典》划分为21册，总计收载文物5000余件。对每件文物的描述，除质地、规格、馆藏等基本要素外，重点描述其在民生健康中的作用。对少数暂不明确的事项在括号中注明待考。对引自各博物馆的材料除在文物后列出馆藏外，还在书后再次统一列出馆名或参考书目，以充分尊重其馆藏权，也同时维护本典作者的引用权。

21世纪，围绕人类健康的生命科学将飞速发展，但科学离不开文化，文化离不开文物。发掘文物承载的信息为现实服务，谨引用横渠先生四言之两语："为天地立心，为生民立命"，既作为编撰本《图典》之宗旨，也是我们践行国家"一带一路"倡议的具体努力。希冀通过本《图典》的出版发行，教育国人，提振中华民族精神；走向世界，为人类健康事业贡献力量。

李经纬　梁峻　刘学春

2017年6月于北京

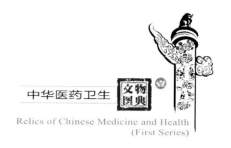

中华医药卫生 文物图典

Relics of Chinese Medicine and Health
(First Series)

目 录

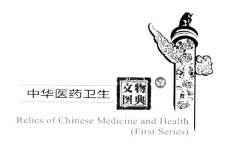
Contents

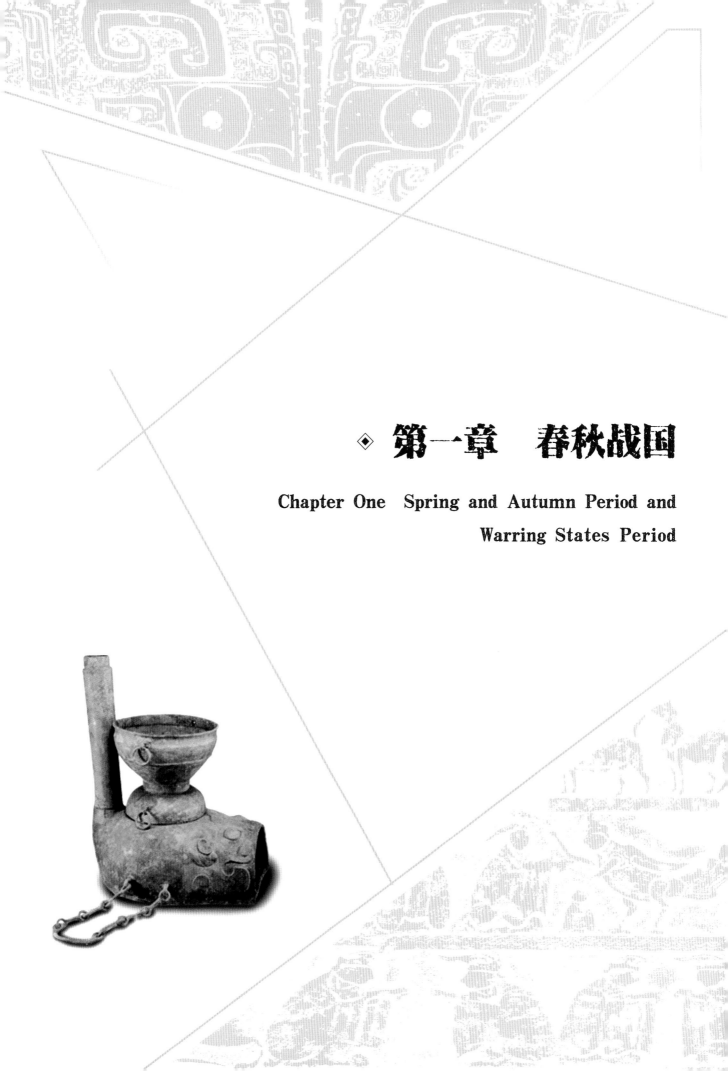

◆ 第一章　春秋战国

Chapter One　Spring and Autumn Period and Warring States Period

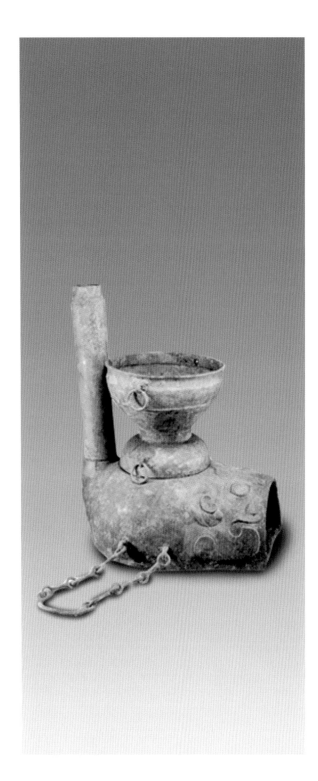

提梁虎形青铜灶

春秋（前 770—前 476）

铜质

通高 160 厘米

Tiger-shaped Bronze Stove with a
Hooped Handle

Spring and Autumn Period (770 B.C.–476 B.C.)

Bronze

Height 160 cm

由灶身、灶具、烟囱几部分构成。此件以子
母口套接的多节烟囱可以控制火力的大小，
可拆装的结构又使形体庞大的灶具能适用军
旅或游牧的需要。这种先进的设计代表了东
周时期炉灶设计的较高水平，实为饮食文化
中不可多得的珍品。山西省太原市金胜村晋
国赵卿墓出土。

山西省考古研究所藏

This stove consists of the stove body, cooking
utensils and the chimney. Chimneys are
connected by two matching mouths to control
heat, and because of its removable structure,
this large sized stove can be applied to military
and nomadic needs. The advanced designing
technique signifies the high level of stove
design in Eastern Zhou Dynasty and the stove
is a treasury of Chinese culinary art. It was
unearthed from tomb of Zhao Qing who lived
in Jin State, Jinsheng Village, Taiyuan City,
Shanxi Province.

Preserved in Shanxi Provincial Institute of Archaeology

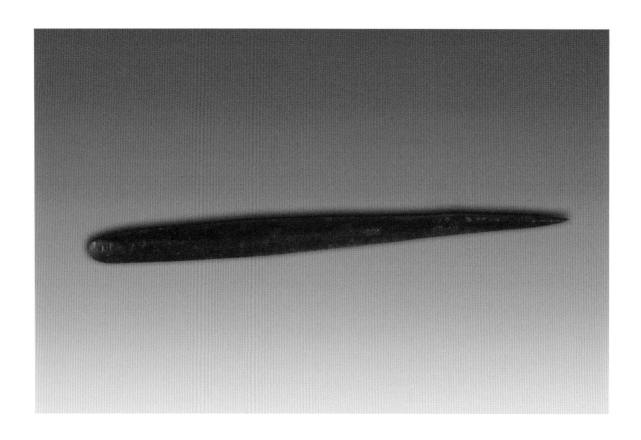

砭针

战国

铜质

长 4.6 厘米，刃宽 0.15 厘米

Flint Needle

Warring States Period

Bronze

Length 4.6 cm/ Width of Blade 0.15 cm

此针一端为针尖，腰呈三棱形；一端为半圆状刃。尖端用以刺病，刃端用以放血。1978 年内蒙古达拉特旗树林召采集。

陕西医史博物馆藏

This three-edged needle has one end as a needle tip for stabbing treatment and another end as a semicircled blade for bloodletting. It was collected from Shulin Zhao, Dalate County, Inner Mongolia, in 1978.

Preserved in Shaanxi Museum of Medical History

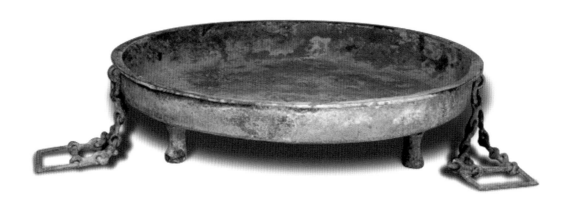

蟠螭纹炉

战国前期

铜质

口径 50.5 厘米，通高 34.5 厘米，重 7.14 千克

Stove with Pan Chi Pattern

Early Warring States Period

Bronze

Mouth Diameter 50.5 cm/ Height 34.5 cm/ Weight 7.14 kg

圆形，似盘，三短足，两侧有环附长链，炉身饰蟠螭纹。炉是古人燎炭取暖的用具，最早约出现于春秋前期。蟠螭纹炉附有铜铲，炉盘内部有铲的锈迹，炉、铲俱全。1954 年入藏。

故宫博物院藏

This stove is round like a tray with three short legs, and attached to long chains on both sides and decorated with the pattern of Pan Chi, a legendary dragon. Stoves, first appearing in early Spring and Autumn Period, were used by the ancients to burn charcoal for heat. The stove is equipped with a bronze shovel and the rust of the shovel can still be found in the stove. Both the stove and the shovel are kept in stock. It was collected in 1954.

Preserved in The Palace Museum

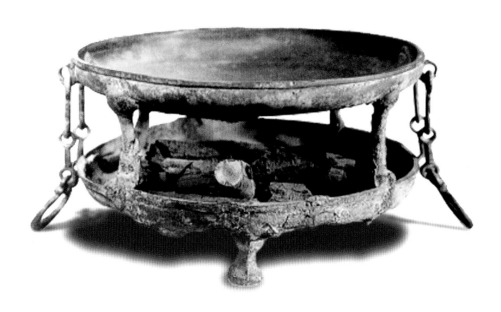

铜炉盘

战国前期

铜质

通高 21.2 厘米

上盘：口径 39.2 厘米

下盘：口径 38.2 厘米

提链：长 20 厘米

Copper Stove Tray

Early Warring States Period

Copper

Height 21.2 cm

Upper Tray: Mouth Diameter 39.2 cm

Lower Tray: Mouth Diameter 38.2 cm

Chains: Length 20 cm

出土时，盘内盛有鱼骨，经鉴定是鲫鱼骨。
盘底有明显的烟炱，而炉盘内尚盛有十几
块未燃尽的木炭。复合烹饪器。湖北省随
州市曾侯乙墓出土。

湖北省博物馆藏

When the stove tray was unearthed, fish
bones were founded inside the tray, which
were identified to be from the crucian carp.
There is soot left on the bottom of the tray
and there was a dozen of pieces of unburnt
charcoal inside the stove. It is a composite
cooking vessel, unearthed in Zeng Marquis
Yi Tomb of Warring States of Suizhou City,
Hubei Province.
Preserved in Hubei Provincial Museum

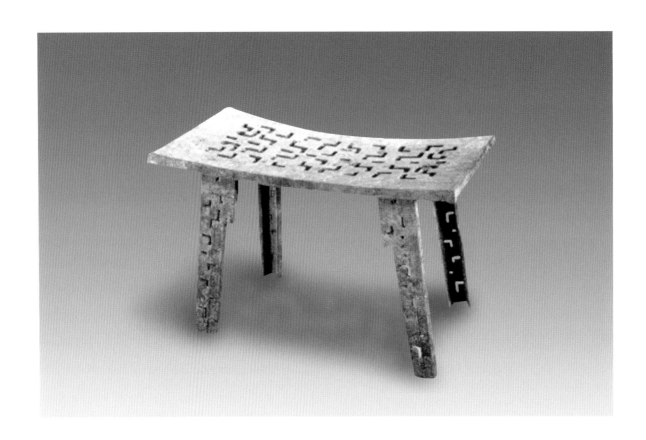

青铜俎

春秋后期

铜质

长 35.5 厘米，宽 21 厘米，通高 24 厘米

Bronze Zu

Late Spring and Autumn Period

Bronze

Length 35.5 cm/ Width 21 cm/ Height 24 cm

按照周礼的规定，俎也是祭祀礼器的一种，其使用介于镬鼎、升鼎和豆之间，是承载、切割肉食的器具。河南省淅川县下寺楚墓出土。

河南博物院藏

According to the ritual of Zhou Dynasty, "Zu" was a sacrificial vessel and its function falls within tripod caldron, Sheng Tripod and Dou Tripod and it was used to hold or chop meat served as sacrifices. It was unearthed from Chu Tomb, Xiasi Village, Xichuan County, Henan Province.

Preserved in Henan Museum

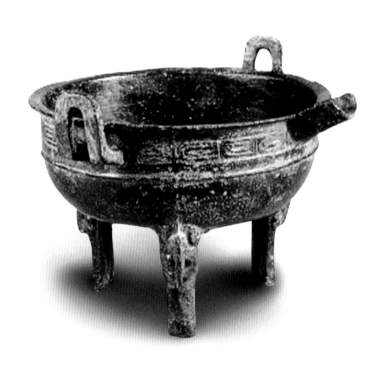

青铜带流鼎

春秋前期

铜质

口径 15 厘米，高 12.4 厘米

Bronze Tripod with a Spout

Early Spring and Autumn Period

Bronze

Mouth Diameter 15 cm/ Height 12.4 cm

此件在宽扁的口沿上斜向伸出了一支流，使煮食的鼎自身又有了倾倒羹汁的功能。商周青铜鼎中有流的较少见。另外，腹两侧的方形中空耳也不像立耳那样直立于口沿上，而是自鼎腹一侧横向伸出后再直立起来，故称之为"附耳"。附耳是东周青铜器中流行的做法。

北京大学赛克勒考古与艺术博物馆藏

On the edge of the wide flat mouth of the tripod extends obliquely a spout; therefore, the tripod can not only be used as a cooking vessel but can also be used to pour soup and juice. It is rare in Shang and Zhou Dynasties to see a bronze tripod with a spout. In addition, the cuboid hollow ears on both sides of the belly are not like prick ears standing straight on the mouth edge. They extend from the belly vertically and then go up straight. Therefore, they are called "attached prick ears", which are popular additions on bronze tripod in Eastern Zhou Dynasty.

Preserved in Arthur M. Sackler Museum of Art and Archaeology at Peking University

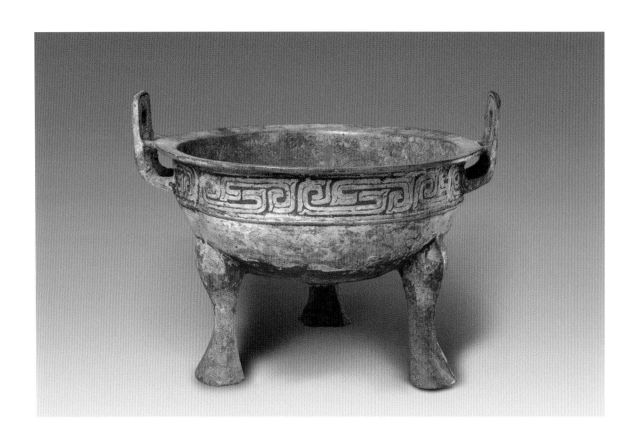

陈侯鼎

春秋前期

铜质

宽 35 厘米，通高 23.6 厘米，重 5.58 千克

Tripod with Characters "Chen Hou"

Early Spring and Autumn Period

Bronze

Width 35 cm/ Height 23.6 cm/ Weight 5.58 kg

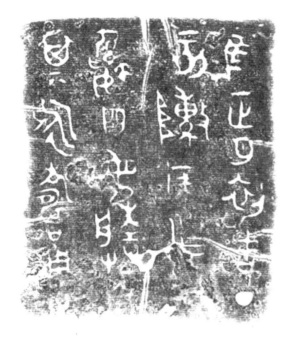

敞口，浅圜腹，马蹄足，口沿外附双耳。颈饰窃曲纹。器内有铭文4行20字，记陈侯为其女□妫四母做陪嫁的鼎，祈望她长寿用之。1958年收购。

故宫博物院藏

The tripod has an open mouth, a shallow round belly and three horseshoe-shaped feet. Two prick ears attached to the outside of the mouth. The neck decorated with Qie Qu pattern There is an inscription of 20 characters in 4 lines inside the tripod saying that this vessel was used as dowry by Chen Hou for her daughter with a wish that she could live a longer life. It was acquired in 1958.
Preserved in The Palace Museum

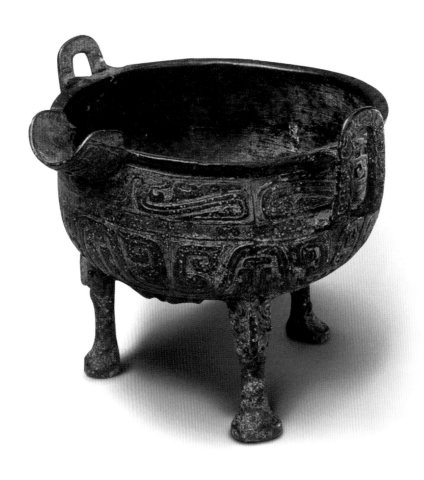

夔纹有流鼎

春秋前期

铜质

宽 21.1 厘米，通高 15.5 厘米，重 1.52 千克

此鼎的造型较为特殊。圆腹，圜底，三蹄足。二附耳，耳上方有平行二柱，柱另一端与鼎口相铸接。鼎口上还置一半圆形流，可用来倾倒汁液用。颈部饰垂冠顾首的夔龙纹，腹上饰环带纹，并均以云雷纹为地纹。三兽上端饰浮雕兽面纹，中置扉棱。1946 年入藏。

故宫博物院藏

Tripod with Kui Pattern and a Spout

Early Spring and Autumn Period

Bronze

Width 21.1 cm/ Height 15.5 cm/ Weight 1.52 kg

With a special design, the tripod has a round belly, a round bottom, three horseshoe-shaped feet and two prick ears on which stand two parallel pillars. One end of the pillar is connected with the mouth on which there is a semicircular spout for discharging juice. The neck is decorated with a pattern of Kui-dragon looking back with its head hanging down, a legendary dragon. The belly is decorated with ring-ribbon-like pattern and with cloud and thunder patterns as the background pattern. On the upper part of the three dragons, there are animal faces in relief pattern and in the middle there are ridges. It was collected in 1946.

Preserved in The Palace Museum

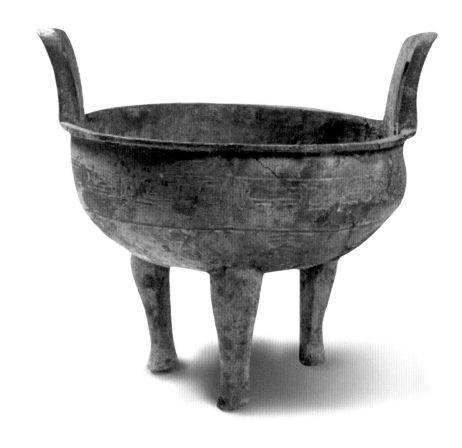

青铜变形窃曲纹鼎

春秋中期

铜质

口径 35.5 厘米，通高 33 厘米

直耳微侈，半球形浅腹，圜底，三蹄足上粗下细，腹饰窃曲纹一道，下有一条弦纹。高淳区青山公社出土。

镇江博物馆藏

Bronze Tripod with Deformed Qie Qu Pattern

Mid Spring and Autumn Period

Bronze

Mouth Diameter 35.5 cm/ Height 33 cm

The tripod has two slightly larger straight ears on it, a hemispherical shallow belly, a round bottom and three horseshoe-shaped feet which are thick in the upper part and thin in the lower part. The belly is decorated with a ring of Qie Qu Pattern under which there is a string pattern. It was unearthed from Qingshan Commune, Gaochun District.

Preserved in Zhenjiang Municipal Museum

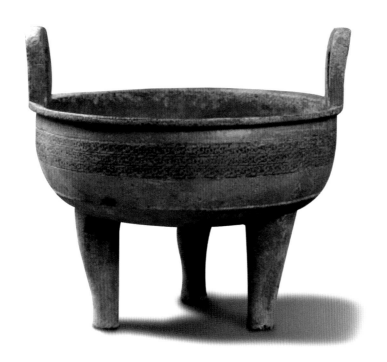

蟠虺纹鼎

春秋中期

铜质

口径 33 厘米，高 29 厘米

Tripod with Pan Hui Pattern

Mid Spring and Autumn Period

Bronze

Mouth Diameter 33 cm/ Height 29 cm

宽平缘外折，方唇，立耳厚大，略向外撇，腹呈盆形，较浅，底近平，足为简化的兽蹄形，上粗下细。腹部饰三周细密的蟠虺纹。此鼎造型轻巧，装饰简洁，为吴国地区青铜器中的精品。

南京市博物馆藏

The wide and flat edge is folded outward. The tripod has a square lip and thick prick ears slightly inclining outward. The shallow belly is basin-shaped with flat bottom and the feet are in simplified horseshoe-like shape with thick upper part and thin lower part. The belly is decorated with three circles of dense Pan Hui pattern. The tripod, with light design and simple decor, is a boutique of bronze vessels in Wu State region.

Preserved in Nanjing Municipal Museum

王子午鼎（附匕）

春秋

青铜质

口径 62 厘米，通高 62 厘米

Tripod Belonging to Wang Ziwu〔with a Dagger〕

Spring and Autumn Period

Bronze

Mouth Diameter 62 cm/ Height 62 cm

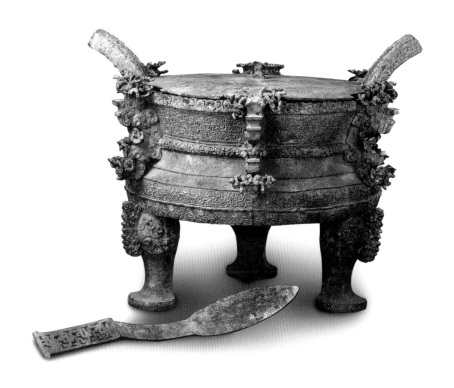

侈口，立耳外撇，束腰，鼓腹，平底，兽首蹄足；上有平盖，顶铸桥纽。匕如柳叶，柄部镂空。器身有六怪兽，昂首卷尾，举喙附壁。器表饰浅浮雕蟠螭纹、窃曲纹和垂鳞纹。器内壁及底部有铭文 84 字。大意为：王子午自铸铜鼎，以祭先祖文王和进行盟祀；我施人民以德政，因而受到尊重，望子孙后代以我为准绳。1978 年河南省淅川下寺 2 号楚墓出土。

河南博物院藏

The tripod has a large mouth, two attached prick ears inclining outward, a tightened waist, a swelling belly, a flat bottom, three hoof-like feet and a flat cover on which there is a bridge-like knob. The dagger is in the shape of willow leaf with a hollow handle. There is a design of 6 beasts lifting up their heads and curling up tails attached on the body and the edge of the tripod. The surface of the tripod is decorated with shallow relief of Pan Chi pattern, Qie Qu patterns, and vertical scales. There is an inscription of 84 characters on the inner wall and the bottom of the vessel which roughly means that "The bronze tripod was made by Wang Ziwu as a sacrificial vessel to worship ancestor King Wen and for alliance. I (Wang Ziwu) rule people by moral means thus I receive people's respect, so I hope I can be the criterion for my later generations". It was unearthed in the No.2 Chu tomb, Xiasi Village, Xichuan County, Henan Province, in 1978.

Preserved in Henan Museum

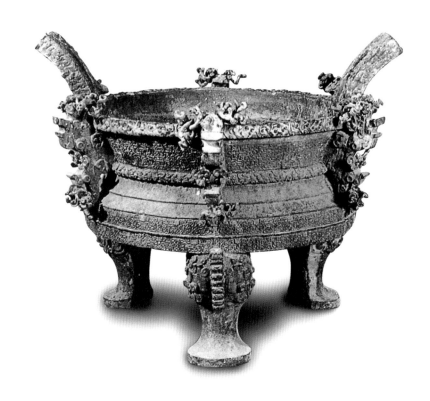

王子午升鼎

春秋

青铜质

口径 66 厘米，通高 68 厘米

Sheng Tripod Belonging to Wang Ziwu

Spring and Autumn Period

Bronze

Mouth Diameter 66 cm/ Height 68 cm

此鼎外部装饰繁缛细致，纤巧奇诡，系商周以来中原青铜文化与楚人诡丽巧思的完美结合体；其装饰性与实用性亦有机统一。此鼎属楚庄王之子——楚康王时的大臣子庚所有，他所任官职是令尹，故此鼎又称令尹子庚鼎。河南省淅川县下寺楚墓出土。

河南博物院藏

The tripod, decorated with elaborate and delicate patterns, dainty and unique, is a perfect combination of the bronze culture of the Central Plains of China, and the ingenuity of Chu people since Shang and Zhou Dynasties. It integrates decorative and pragmatic functions. The tripod belonged to Zi Geng, minister of King Kang of Chu's era who is the son of King Zhuang of Chu State, Zi Geng was at that time the prime minister of the state; therefore, the tripod is also called "Tripod for Prime Minister Zi Geng". It was unearthed from Chu tomb, Xiasi Village, Xichuan County, Henan Province. Preserved in Henan Museum

蔡子鼎

春秋后期

铜质

口径 23 厘米，宽 28.2 厘米，通高 33 厘米，重 6.77 千克

Tripod Belonging to Cai Zi

Late Spring and Autumn Period

Bronze

Mouth Diameter 23 cm/ Width 28.2 cm/ Height 33 cm/ Weight 6.77 kg

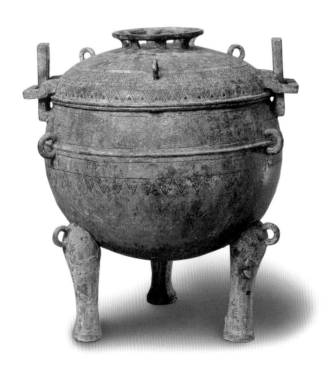

器身连盖近球形。盖上有透空圆形捉手；盖、腹、足相对应铸有小环，能用绳穿系；附耳直；下具三个兽蹄足。通饰变形的蟠虺纹和三角纹。盖上铸有 5 字铭文。1959 年收购。

故宫博物院藏

The whole body of the tripod is spherical with a round hollow knob on its cover, and small hoops on the cover, the belly and the feet so that they can tether through a rope. The tripod, with prick ears and three horseshoe-shaped feet, is decorated with disformed Pan Hui patterns and triangle patterns. There is an inscription of 5 characters on the cover. The tripod was acquired in 1959.

Preserved in The Palace Museum

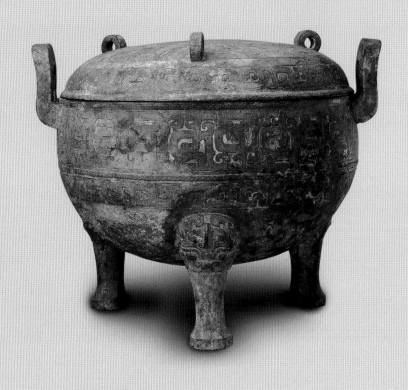

蟠虺纹鼎

春秋后期

青铜质

宽 55.5 厘米，通高 45 厘米，重 24.56 千克

Tripod with Pan Hui Pattern

Late Spring and Autumn Period

Bronze

Width 55.5 cm/ Height 45 cm/ Weight 24.56 kg

大腹，圆底，蹄形足。有盖，盖饰三环纽和三道蟠虺纹；双附耳，耳两面饰蟠虺纹，两侧饰回纹；腹饰二道蟠虺纹，间以绳纹；足饰兽面纹。1958 年 9 月收购。

故宫博物院藏

The tripod has a big belly, a round bottom, three horseshoe-shaped feet, a cover and two prick ears. The cover has a decor of three ring-like knobs and three rings of Pan Hui pattern. Two larger sides of the ears are decorated with Pan Hui pattern while two smaller sides are decorated with rectangular spiral pattern. The belly is covered with two rings of Pan Hui pattern between which there is rope pattern while the legs are decorated with animal mask pattern. The tripod was acquired in September 1958.

Preserved in The Palace Museum

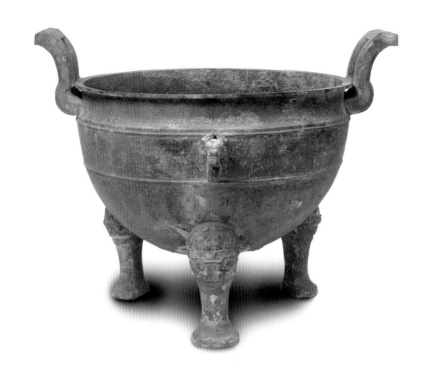

蟠虺纹大鼎

春秋后期

青铜质

口径 77 厘米，宽 102 厘米，通高 75 厘米，重 64.2 千克

Large Tripod with Pan Hui Pattern

Late Spring and Autumn Period

Bronze

Mouth Diameter 77 cm/ Width 102 cm/ Height 75 cm/ Weight 64.2 kg

圆鼎，侈口，有附耳，圆底，蹄形足。腹前后有环，环上饰兽头。颈敛，饰重环纹、蟠虺纹、三角纹；腹饰上、下二道绳纹，间饰以蟠虺纹，下垂蕉叶纹；足饰兽面纹。1923 年河南新郑出土，1956 年国家文物局调拨。

故宫博物院藏

The tripod has a round body, a large mouth, two prick ears, a round bottom, and horseshoe-shaped feet. Knobs, with a decoration of pattern of the beast head, are on the front and back sides of the belly. The neck is converged with double ring pattern, Pan Hui pattern and triangle pattern. The belly has two rings of rope pattern on the upper part and the lower part respectively, between which there is decor of Pan Hui pattern under which there is the pattern of drooped banana leaves. There are animal mask patterns on the feet. The tripod was unearthed from Xinzheng City, Henan Province, in 1923, and allocated from State Administration of Cultural Heritage in 1956.
Preserved in The Palace Museum

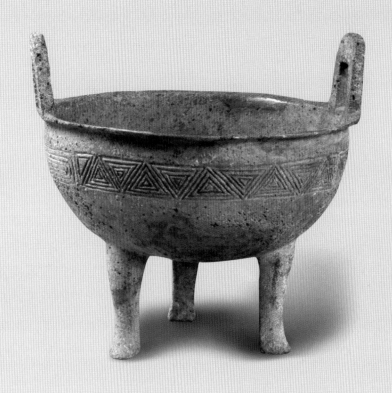

铜鼎

春秋

铜质

口径 23.1 厘米，高 21.6 厘米

Copper Tripod

Spring and Autumn Period

Copper

Mouth Diameter 23.1 cm/ Height 21.6 cm

平沿外折，方唇，立耳，半球形腹，圆底，下具三条兽蹄足，排列内聚，腹部饰一周龙纹。南京市浦口长山子出土。

南京市博物馆藏

The tripod has an edge folded outward, a square mouth, two prick ears, a hemispherical belly, a round bottom and three close gathered hoof-like feet. The belly is decorated with a circle of dragon patterns. It was unearthed from Chang Shanzi, Pukou District, Nanjing City. Preserved in Nanjing Municipal Museum

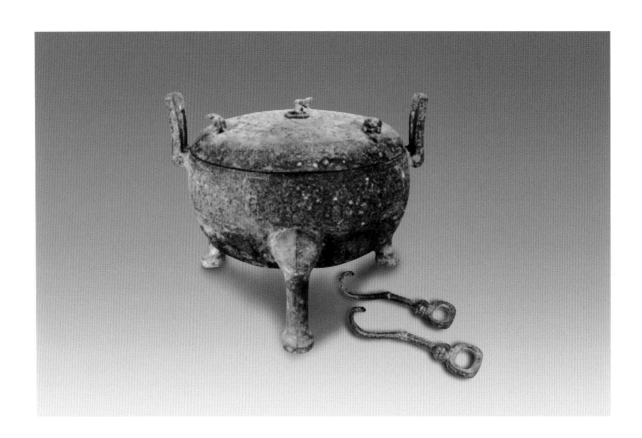

曾侯乙镬鼎

战国前期

青铜质

口径 57.4 厘米，通高 57 厘米，重 41 千克

Huo Tripod Belonging to Marquis Yi of Zeng State

Early Warring States Period

Bronze

Mouth Diameter 57.4 cm/ Height 57 cm/ Weight 41 kg

鼎最初的作用是煮食，但商周时期的青铜鼎分化出了专以烹煮牲肉的镬鼎和专以盛装熟肉并调味的升鼎。周礼又将这种分工加以规范，升鼎成为祭祀的重心而称为"正鼎"，保存了原始功能的镬鼎却成为陪鼎。此鼎出土时，腹腔内盛有半个牛体，腹底残留有烟熏火烧的痕迹。湖北省随州市曾侯乙墓出土。

湖北省博物馆藏

Tripods were originally used as cooking vessels; however, in Shang and Zhou Dynasties, bronze tripods were divided into two main categories: one type refers to "Huo" tripods used for cooking meat and the other type refers to "Sheng" tripods for containing and seasoning the cooked meat. The ritual of Zhou Dynasty regulated the division by making "Sheng" tripods as the core sacrificial vessels, thus called main tripods, and "Huo" tripods which preserved the primary use as accessory tripods, the accompanying tripods. When the tripod was unearthed, half of the body of an ox was found inside the vessel and there still remained traces of smoke and fire on the bottom. It was unearthed in Zeng Marquis Yi Tomb of Warring States of Suizhou City, Hubei Province.

Preserved in Hubei Provincial Museum

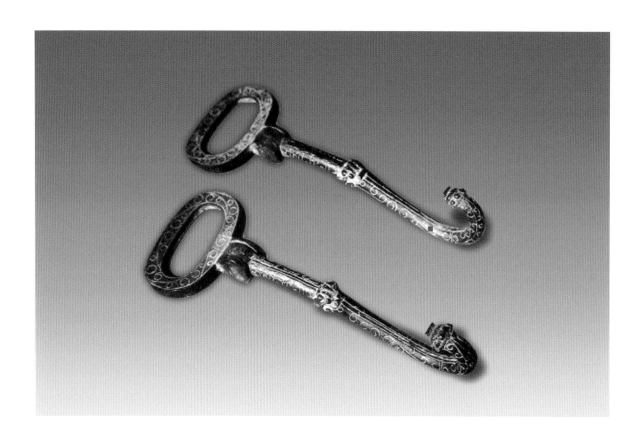

青铜鼎钩

Bronze Hooks for Bronze Tripod

战国前期

青铜质

通长 24.4 厘米

钩距：5.8 厘米

提环：长 9 厘米，宽 5.3 厘米

Early Warring Stated Period

Bronze

Length 24.4 cm

Distance Between Two Hooks: 5.8 cm

Haul Loop: Length 9 cm/ Width 5.3 cm

此对鼎钩属于一件牛形盖大鼎，出土时放在鼎盖上，分为提手和弯钩两部分。这类铜钩装饰华美，铸造精美，设计也较为先进独到。钩身背面有鸟篆铭文"曾侯乙作持用终"7字。

湖北省博物馆藏

This pair of hooks belongs to a tripod with a large ox-shaped cover. When they were unearthed, they were found on the cover of the tripod and divided into two parts, haul loops and hooks. This kind of bronze hooks has a beautiful decoration, exquisite, advance and unique design. There is an inscription of 7 characters in bird seal script on the back of the hooks.

Preserved in Hubei Provincial Museum

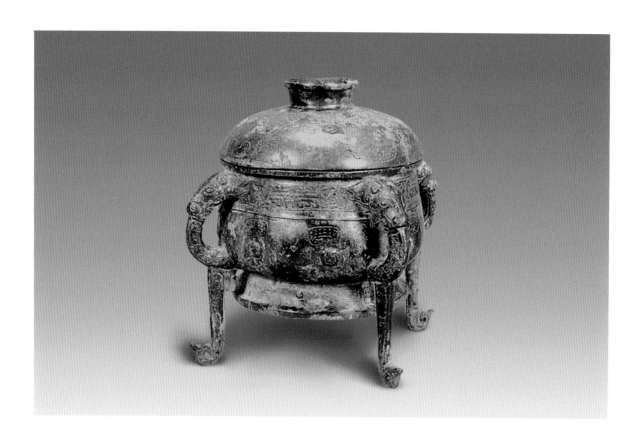

曾侯乙升鼎

战国早期

青铜质

口径 45.8 厘米，底径 42.1 厘米，通高 35.5 厘米

Sheng Tripod Belonging to Marquis Yi of Zeng State

Early Warring States Period

Bronze

Mouth Diameter 45.8 cm/ Bottom Diameter 42.1 cm/ Height 35.5 cm

此鼎为典型的楚式风格，造型生动。线槽内原镶嵌有绿松石等装饰物，现已脱落。湖北省随州市曾侯乙墓出土。

湖北省博物馆藏

The tripod displays a typical style of the tripods of the Chu State. Decorations like turquoises are inlaid inside the trunk but are lost now. It was unearthed in Zeng Marquis Yi Tomb of Warring States of Suizhou City, Hubei Province.

Preserved in Hubei Provincial Museum

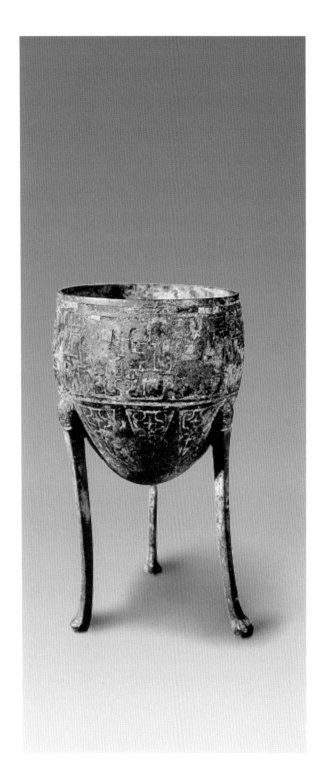

青铜鼎形器

战国早期

青铜质

口径 11.8 厘米，通高 20.7 厘米，腹深 11.5 厘米

Bronze Tripod-shaped Vessel

Early Warring States Period

Bronze

Mouth Diameter 11.8 cm/ Height 20.7 cm/ Belly
Depth 11.5 cm

直口，深腹，腹底下垂，有三条瘦长的蹄形足。器表铸出纹饰：口部和腹中部各有一周凹弦纹将纹样分成两组，上部为勾连卷云纹，下部为垂叶纹，足根为兽面纹，蹄面饰卷云纹。在凹弦纹及勾连卷云纹的凹槽内，原曾镶嵌绿松石，大多现已脱落。鼎身与三足是分铸成型后焊接为一体的。湖北省随州市曾侯乙墓出土。

湖北省博物馆藏

The vessel has a straight mouth, a deep sagging belly, and three thin and long hoof-shaped feet. The surface of the vessel is covered by patterns. Two circles of concave string pattern on the mouth and on the middle part of the belly respectively divide patterns into two groups; on the upper part there is cloud-like patterns while the lower is decorated with drooping leaf pattern and the heels are decorated with animal mask patterns while on the feet there are cloud-like patterns. Turquoises were originally embedded in the groove between the concave string pattern and the cloud-like pattern, but most of them are lost now. The body and the three legs are separately made and then welded as a whole. It was unearthed in Zeng Marquis Yi Tomb of Warring States of Suizhou City, Hubei Province.

Preserved in Hubei Provincial Museum

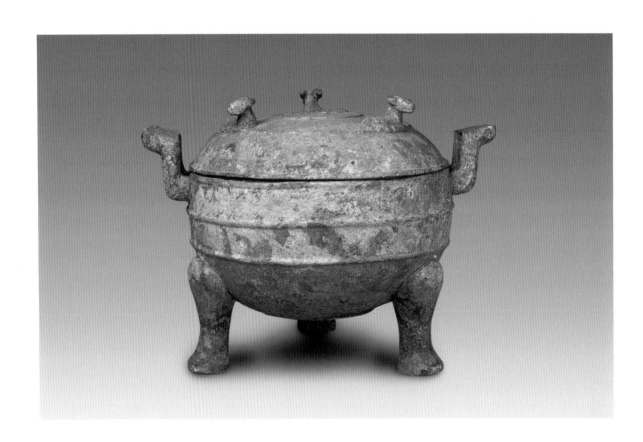

单孝子鼎

战国前期

青铜质

口径 21 厘米，宽 31.8 厘米，通高 23.6 厘米，重 4.64 千克

Shan Xiaozi Tripod

Early Warring States Period

Bronze

Mouth Diameter 21 cm/ Width 31.8 cm/ Height 23.6 cm/ Weight 4.64 kg

圆体，三蹄形足，双附耳，有盖，盖上饰三牺。器身饰弦纹二周。盖、器对铭，各有铭文 16 字。饪食器。1954 年收购。

故宫博物院藏

The tripod used as a food utensil has a round body, three horseshoe-shaped feet, two prick ears and a cover on which there is a design of three animals. The body is decorated with two circles of string pattern. There is an inscription of 16 characters on the cover and the body respectively. The tripod was acquired in 1954.

Preserved in The Palace Museum

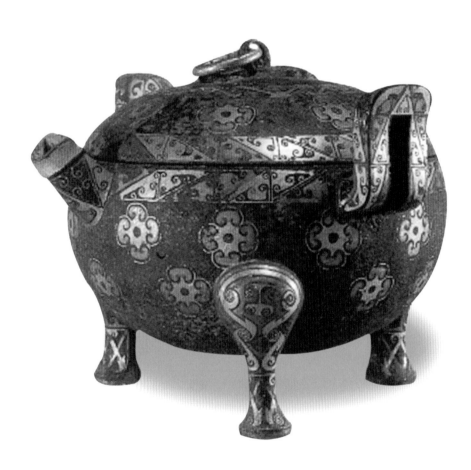

错金银有流铜鼎

战国中晚期

青铜质

口径 10.5 厘米，高 11.4 厘米

此类有流鼎较为少见，是盛装流质食物如肉羹类食品的器具，为东周王室用品。1981 年河南省洛阳市东周王城遗址出土。

洛阳市文物考古研究院藏

Gold and Silver Smeared Bronze Tripod with a Spout

Mid and Late Warring States Period

Bronze

Mouth Diameter 10.5 cm/ Height 11.4 cm

This type of tripods is rarely found. It was used by the royal families of the King of Eastern Zhou Dynasty as a container for fluid food such as bouillon. It was unearthed from the city relics of Eastern Zhou Dynasty, Luoyang City, Henan Province in 1981.

Preserved in Luoyang City Cultural Relics and Archaeology Research Institute

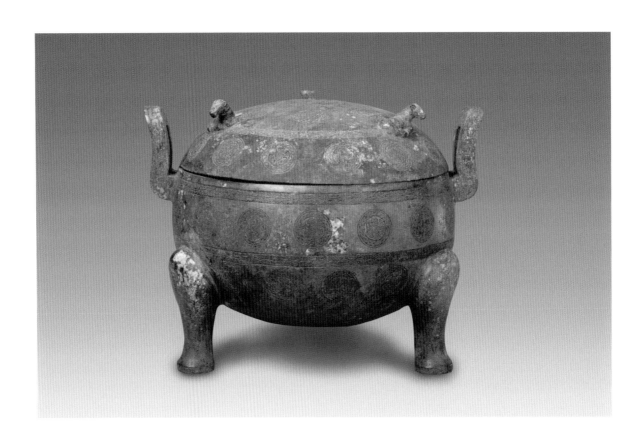

团花纹鼎

战国后期

青铜质

口径 17.9 厘米，宽 25.8 厘米，通高 18.2 厘米，重 3.8 千克

Tripod with Pattern of Clusters of Flowers

Late Warring States Period

Bronze

Mouth Diameter 17.9 cm/ Width 25.8 cm/ Height 18.2 cm/ Weight 3.8 kg

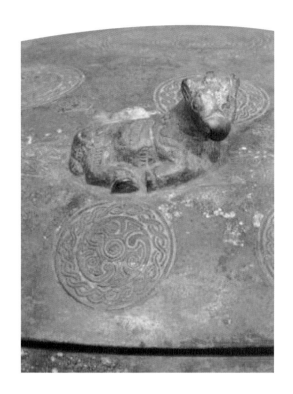

圆体，三足，双附耳，有盖，盖上饰三伏牺。三牺间以回纹相连，内、外各饰团花一周；器身饰回纹、团花纹各二周；附耳两面饰回纹，两侧饰双夔纹。清宫旧藏。

故宫博物院藏

The tripod has a round body, three legs, two attached prick ears and a cover which is decorated with the pattern of three crouched animals that are connected with rectangular spiral pattern. On both the inner and the outer sides of the rectangular spiral pattern there are circles of pattern of clusters of flowers. The body is covered with two circles of rectangular spiral pattern and pattern of clusters of flowers while the attached prick ears have fret pattern on both the larger sides and the two designs of Kui-dragon on both smaller sides. It used to serve the imperial palace in Qing Dynasty.

Preserved in The Palace Museum

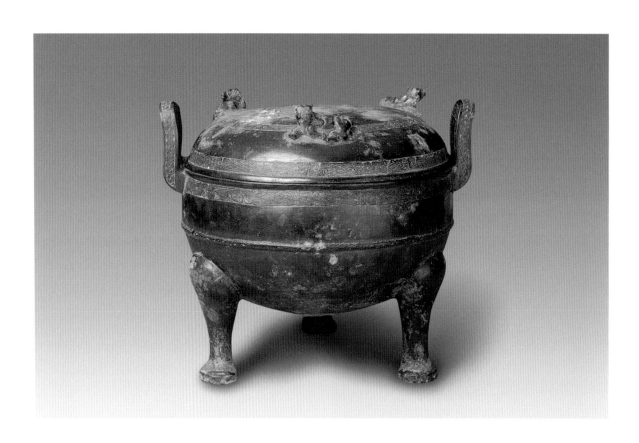

三牺鼎

战国后期

青铜质

宽 23.3 厘米，通高 19.9 厘米，重 2.84 千克

Tripod with Designs of Three Animals

Late Warring States Period

Bronze

Width 23.3 cm/ Height 19.9 cm/ Weight 2.84 kg

圆体，三蹄形足，双附耳，有盖，盖上饰
三卧牺，腹部有凸棱一周。盖、颈、耳部
均饰有蟠螭纹。1960 年收购。

故宫博物院藏

The tripod has a round body, three hoof-like
feet, two prick ears and a cover decorated
with three crouched animals. The belly has a
circle of raised ridge, and there are Pan Chi
patterns on the cover, the neck and the ears.
The tripod was acquired in 1960.
Preserved in The Palace Museum

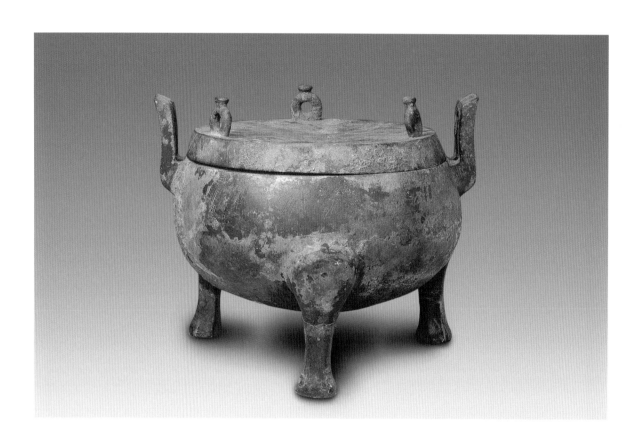

魏鼎

战国后期

青铜质

宽 30.4 厘米，通高 24.2 厘米，重 7.06 千克

Wei Tripod

Late Warring States Period

Bronze

Width 30.4 cm/ Height 24.2 cm/ Weight 7.06 kg

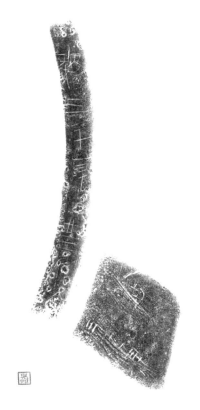

圆体，敛口，三蹄形足，双附耳，有盖，盖上饰三环纽，器口、腹、盖上均有铭文19字，分别记重量和容量。黄镜涵先生捐献。

故宫博物院藏

The tripod has a round body, a converged mouth, three hoof-like feet, two prick ears and a cover decorated with three ring-like knobs. There is an inscription of 19 characters on the mouth, belly and cover recording the weight and volume of the tripod. It was donated to the Museum by Mr. Huang Jinghan.

Preserved in The Palace Museum

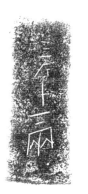

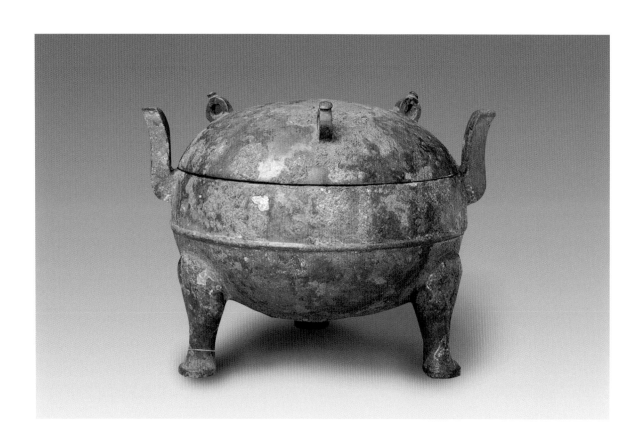

三十五年虒令鼎

战国后期

青铜质

宽 27.4 厘米，通高 19.2 厘米，重 4.27 千克

Si County Magistrate Tripod Forged in 35th Year

Late Warring States Period

Bronze

Width 27.4 cm/ Height 19.2 cm/ Weight 4.27 kg

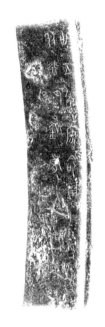

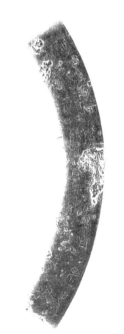

圆体，三蹄形足，双附耳，有盖，盖上饰
三纽，器腹饰一周凸棱。盖、器各有铭文
18 字，对铭。1959 年收购。

故宫博物院藏

The tripod has a round body, three hoof-like
feet, two prick ears and a cover decorated
with three knobs. There is a ring of raised
ridge on the belly. There is an inscription of
18 characters in couplet on the cover and the
body respectively. The tripod was acquired
in 1959.

Preserved in The Palace Museum

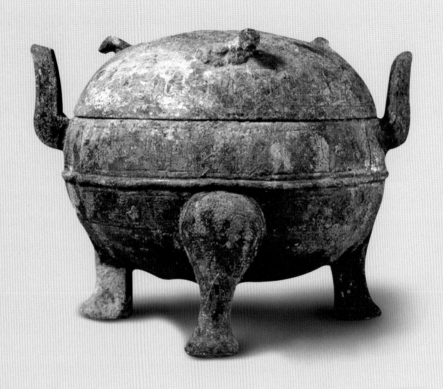

蟠螭纹鼎

战国后期

青铜质

宽 27.5 厘米，通高 21.5 厘米，重 4.63 千克

Tripod with Pan Chi Pattern

Late Warring States Period

Bronze

Width 27.5 cm/ Height 21.5 cm/ Weight 4.63 kg

圆形，大腹，三足，双附耳，有盖。腹饰
蟠螭纹二周。盖上有三伏牺，另饰有蟠螭
纹三周，耳两侧饰鸟纹。河南洛阳西宫秦
墓出土。1956 年国家文物局调拨。

故宫博物院藏

The tripod is round in shape, with a large
belly, three legs, two prick ears and a cover.
The belly is decorated with two rings of Pan
Chi pattern while the cover has a design
of three animals and three rings of Pan
Chi pattern. There is bird pattern on both
sides of the ears. The tripod was unearthed
in Qin tomb of West Palace in Luoyang,
Henan Province, and allocated from State
Administration of Cultural Heritage in 1956.
Preserved in The Palace Museum

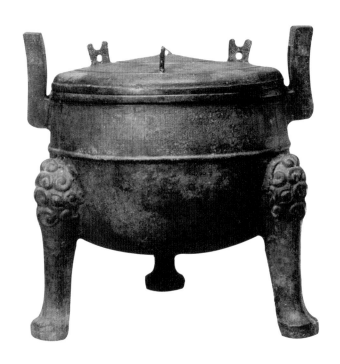

楚王酓胐鼎

战国后期

青铜质

口径 46.6 厘米，宽 60.5 厘米，通高 59.7 厘米，重 53.8 千克

Tripod Forged by King of Chu State Yan Fei

Late Warring States Period

Bronze

Mouth Diameter 46.4 cm/ Width 60.5 cm/ Height 59.7 cm/ Weight 53.8 kg

体圆，三蹄形足，双附耳，有盖，盖上有三短足，盖正中一纽凸起可穿环。附耳、盖与鼎身饰细碎蟠虺纹，足上端饰兽首。盖内、外与器口沿三处刻有铭文。1933年安徽寿县朱家集出土。1954年国家文物局调拨。

故宫博物院藏

The tripod has a round body, three hoof-like feet, two prick ears and a cover on which there are three short legs and a raised pierced knob on the center which can tether the rings. Both the cover and the body are decorated with fine Pan Hui pattern while the feet are decorated with the design of the animal head. There are inscriptions on the inner and the outer side of the cover as well as the mouth edge. It was unearthed in Zhujiaji, Shouxian County, Anhui Province in 1933, and allocated from State Administration of Cultural Heritage in 1954.

Preserved in The Palace Museum

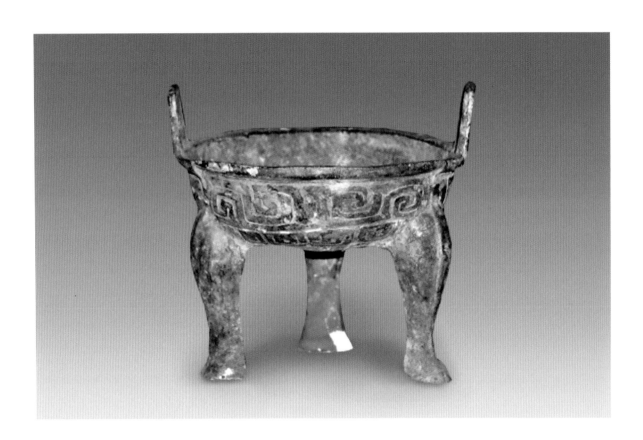

铜鼎

战国

铜质

口径 13 厘米，底径 8.5 厘米，通高 12 厘米，重 0.7 千克

Copper Tripod

Warring States Period

Copper

Mouth Diameter 13 cm/ Bottom Diameter 8.5 cm/ Height 12 cm/ Weight 0.7 kg

平口，斜腹，立耳，三兽足，腹上雕有夔
纹、窃曲纹。礼器，炊器。一足有修补。
20 世纪 70 年代入藏。陕西省西安市鄠邑
区征集。

陕西医史博物馆藏

The tripod has a flat mouth, an oblique belly
decorated with the pattern of Kui-dragon
and Qie Qu pattern, two prick ears and three
hoofed feet, one of which has been repaired.
It was used as a sacrificial and cooking vessel.
It was collected from Huyi District, Xi'an,
Shaanxi Province in 1970s.

Preserved in Shaanxi Museum of Medical History

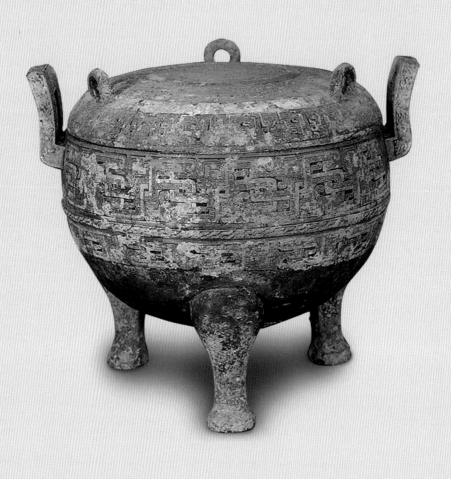

蟠螭纹铜鼎

战国

青铜质

通高 31.5 厘米

器带盖，盖顶有三个饰蟠螭纹的环形纽。鼓腹，两附耳微外撇，圜底，蹄形足。腹饰蟠螭纹，靠下部有一周凸弦纹。

河北博物院藏

Copper Tripod with Pan Chi Pattern

Warring States Period

Bronze

Height 31.5 cm

The tripod has a cover on which there are three ring-like knobs with the pattern of Pan Chi patterns, a swelling belly, two prick ears slight inclining outward, a round bottom and three hoofed feet. The belly is decorated with the pattern of Pan Chi patterns and a circle of convex string pattern on the lower part.

Preserved in Hebei Museum

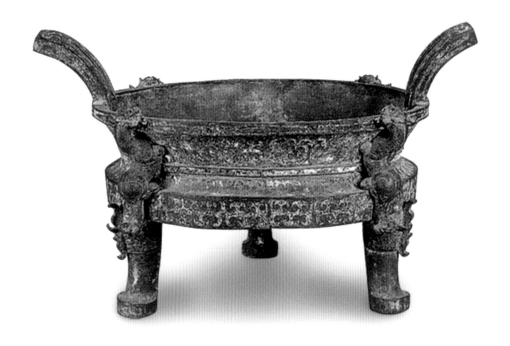

铜升鼎

战国

青铜质

口径 45.8 厘米，通高 35.5 厘米

Copper Sheng Tripod

Warring States Period

Bronze

Mouth Diameter 45.8 cm/ Height 35.5 cm

侈口，立耳外撇，颈内收，束腰，平底。鼎上铭文"升鼎"，器身满饰纹饰，腹壁等距离装饰4只爬兽。

湖北省博物馆藏

The tripod has a wide flared mouth, vertical ears that stand outward, convergent neck, and beam waist, rectangular bottom. There is inscription of the characters "升鼎"（Sheng Ding）and other patterns on the tripod. There are four crawling animals that are arranged with equal distance between one and another.

Preserved in Hubei Provincial Museum

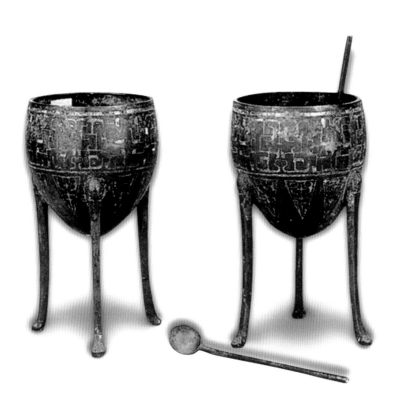

鼎形器

战国

青铜质

左：口径 11.8 厘米，高 20.6 厘米

右：口径 11.4 厘米，高 20.7 厘米

Tripod-shaped Vessel

Warring States Period

Bronze

Left: Mouth Diameter 11.8 cm/ Height 20.6 cm

Right: Mouth Diameter 11.4 cm/ Height 20.7 cm

两件，出土时器内各置长柄铜匕一个。直口，深腹，腹底下垂，有三条瘦长的蹄形足。器表铸出纹饰：口部和腹中部各有一周凹弦纹将纹样分成两组，上部为勾连卷云纹，下部为垂叶纹，足根为兽面纹，蹄面饰卷云纹。在凹弦纹及勾连卷云纹的凹槽内，原曾镶嵌绿松石，大多现已脱落。鼎身与三足是分铸成型后焊接为一体的。1978 年湖北省随州市曾侯乙墓出土。

湖北省博物馆藏

When unearthed, each of the two vessels has a Long handled copper dagger in it. The vessel has a straight mouth, a deep belly, and three thin and long hoof-shaped feet. The surface of the vessel is covered by patterns. Two circles of concave string pattern on the mouth and on the middle part of the belly respectively divide patterns into two groups; on the upper part there is cloud-like patterns while the lower is decorated with descending leaf pattern and the heels are decorated with animal mask patterns while on the feet there are cloud-like patterns. Turquoises were originally embedded in the groove between the concave string pattern and the cloud-like pattern, but most of them are lost now. The body and the three legs are separately made and then welded as a whole. It was unearthed in Zeng Marquis Yi Tomb of Warring States of Suizhou City, Hubei Province, in 1978.

Preserved in Hubei Provincial Museum

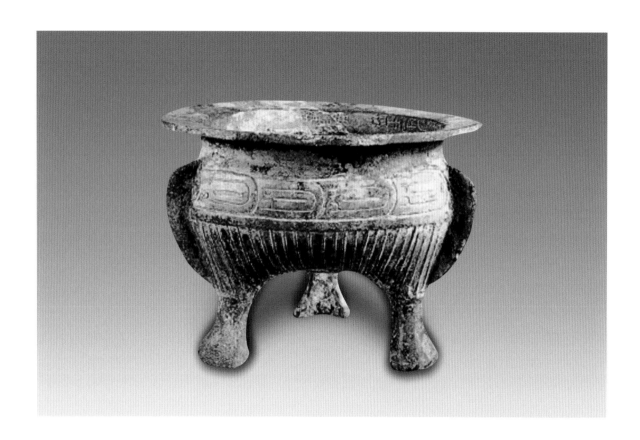

召伯鬲

春秋早期

青铜质

口径 16.5 厘米，高 12 厘米

Zhao Bo Li Tripod

Early Spring and Autumn Period

Bronze

Mouth Diameter 16.5 cm/ Height 12 cm

纵向弦纹装饰是一种较少见的做法。鬲的内壁铸有八字铭文："召白（伯）毛乍（作）王女（汝）尊鬲"，记载了一位名叫毛的贵族为纪念周王对他的恩典及颂扬周王的功德而制作此鬲的史实。文中的"鬲"，作下面正在烧火的高足容器的形象，这是金文中已比较成熟规范的写法，鬲的用途表现得很具体。

北京大学赛克勒考古与艺术博物馆藏

It is rare to see longitudinal string pattern as decoration in bronzes. There is an inscription of 8 Chinese characters on the inner wall of the tripod, meaning that a nobleman named Mao made the tripod in order to commemorate the grace of King of Zhou Dynasty and to praise King's merits. Character "Li" in the inscription is like a long-legged vessel with burning fire under the bottom. It is relatively mature and standard writing in bronze script which specifically shows the usage of Li tripod.
Preserved in Arthur M. Sackler Museum of Art and Archaeology at Peking University

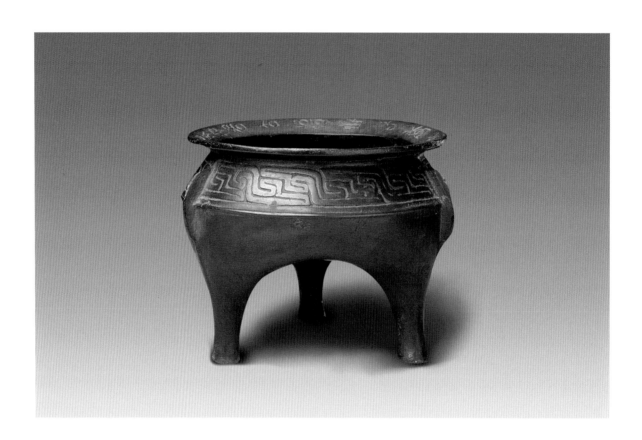

番君鬲

春秋前期

铜质

宽 16 厘米，通高 11.8 厘米，重 1.46 千克

Fan Jun Li Tripod

Early Spring and Autumn Period

Bronze

Width 16 cm/ Height 11.8 cm/ Weight 1.46 kg

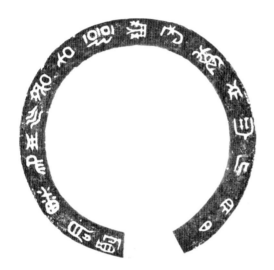

口沿宽且外折，束颈突肩，有凸棱，裆部趋平，足呈兽蹄形。肩饰变形窃曲纹。口沿有铭文 17 字。1964 年入藏。

故宫博物院藏

The tripod has a wide and outward folded mouth edge, a contracted neck, raised shoulder, ridges, flat crotch and hoof-like feet. The shoulder is decorated with deformed Qie Qu patterns. 17 characters were inscribed on the mouth edge. The vessel was collected in 1964.

Preserved in The Palace Museum

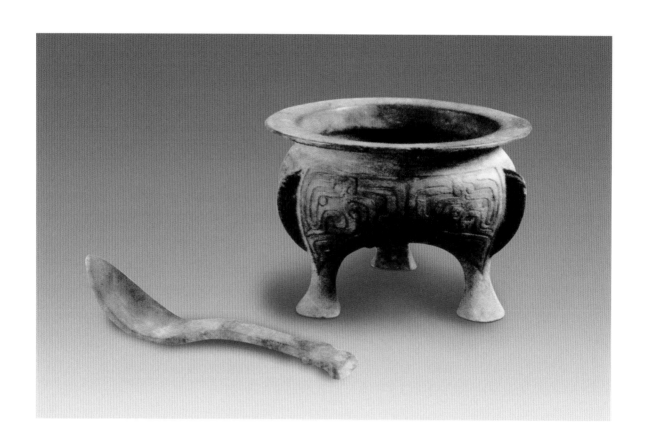

青铜荐鬲

春秋后期前段

铜质

鬲：口径 15.5 厘米，腹径 16.1 厘米，通高 12.6 厘米

匕：长 16 厘米

Bronze Jian Li

Early Phase of Late Spring and Autumn Period

Bronze

Li: Mouth Diameter 15.5 cm/ Belly Diameter 16.1 cm/ Height 12.6 cm

Bi: Length 16 cm

出土时鬲内放置一件青铜短匕，显系与鬲相配的取食工具。口沿上有一周篆书铭文，但起首3字被刮去，存15字，文中说某某自作荐鬲，希望子子孙孙永远传而用之。河南省淅川县下寺楚墓出土。

河南博物院藏

When this Li vessel was unearthed, a bronze Bi (a spoon with shallow elliptical bowl for serving meat and other solids) was found inside it; obviously, it was an accessory tool to the tripod for fetching food. There is a circle of Seal characters on the mouth edge, and 3 of them were scraped off with 15 characters remaining saying that the tripod was made by someone with a wish that it could be used from generation to generation. It was unearthed in the Chu tombs in Xiasi Village, Xichuan County, Henan Province. Preserved in Henan Museum

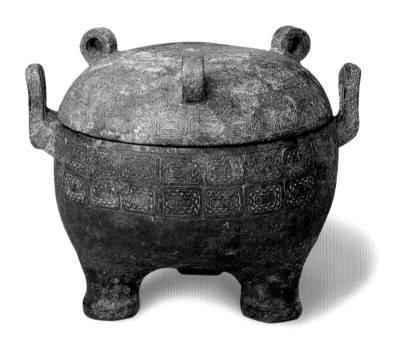

君子之弄鬲

战国前期

铜质

口径 15 厘米，宽 18.4 厘米，通高 14 厘米，重 1.76 千克

Li with Characters "Jun Zi Zhi Nong"

Early Warring States Period

Bronze

Mouth Diameter 15 cm/ Width 18.4 cm/ Height 14 cm/ Weight 1.76 kg

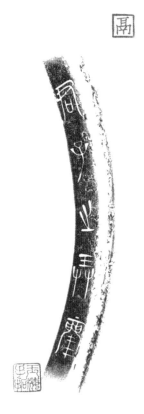

圆体，大腹，三短足，双附耳，有盖，盖上有三环。盖、器各饰有方块绚纹二周，附耳上遍饰花纹。器口沿处有铭文 5 字，记此鬲为君子用于赏玩。河南辉县出土，1958 年收购。

故宫博物院藏

The tripod is round with a large belly, three short legs, two prick ears and a cover on which stand patterns of three rings. Both the cover and the body are decorated with two circles of square twisted rope-like pattern, and two prick ears are covered with patterns. 5 characters were carved on the edge of mouth saying that this tripod was used for appreciation. It was unearthed from Huixian County, Henan Province. It was acquired in 1958.

Preserved in The Palace Museum

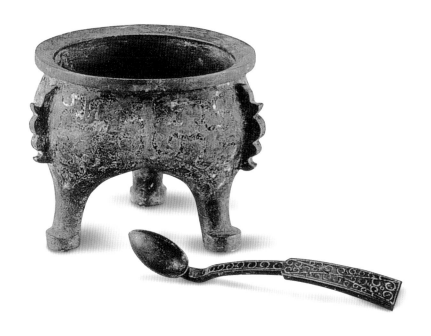

铜小鬲

战国

铜质

口径 15 厘米，通高 12.7 厘米

Small-sized Bronze Li

Warring States Period

Bronze

Mouth Diameter 15 cm/ Height 12.7 cm

食具。敞口微侈，高裆，兽蹄足，器身外壁与鬲足对应处各铸有一道脊棱，有"曾侯乙作持用终"7字铭文。出土时内置长柄小匕。1978年湖北随州市曾侯乙墓出土。

湖北省博物馆藏

The food utensil has a flat and flared mouth, three high hoof-like feet and ridges cast on the belly in the correspondence with the feet of the Li. There are 7 characters meaning "used by Marquis Yi of Zeng". A small knife was found in it when it was unearthed in Zeng Marquis Yi Tomb of Warring States of Suizhou City, Hubei Province, in 1978. Preserved in Hubei Provincial Museum

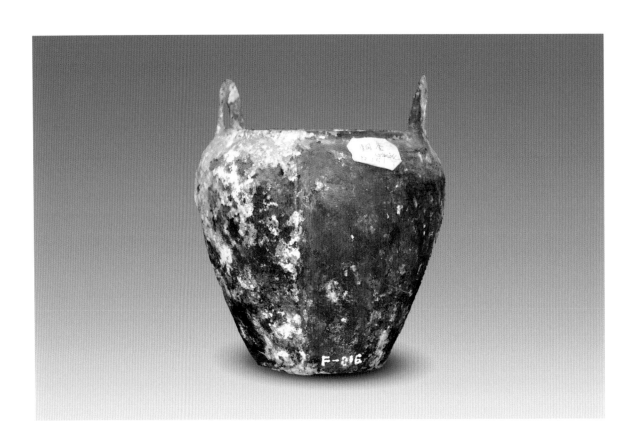

铜釜

战国

铜质

口径 12 厘米，底径 5.5 厘米，通高 6.5 厘米，重 1.25 千克

Copper Fu

Warring States Period

Copper

Mouth Diameter 12 cm/ Bottom Diameter 5.5 cm/ Height 6.5 cm/ Weight 1.25 kg

束口，口上有双耳，圆肩，斜腹，平底，腹部发黑。炊器。完整无损。陕西历史博物馆调拨。

陕西医史博物馆藏

The cauldron has a contracted mouth on which stand two ears. It has a round shoulder, an oblique belly in dark color, a flat bottom. The tripod was used as a cooking vessel and is still in good condition now. It was allocated from Shaanxi History Museum.

Preserved in Shaanxi Museum of Medical History

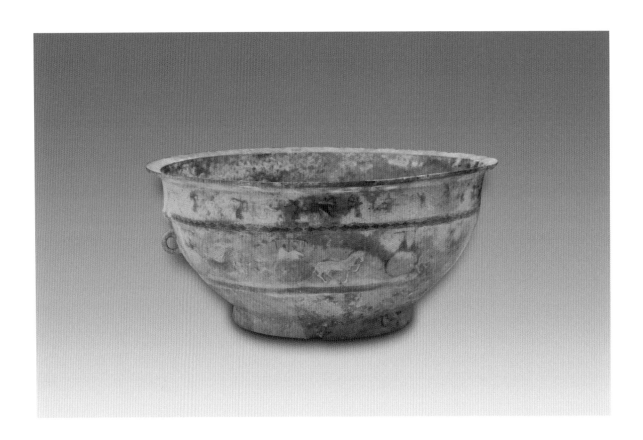

药釜

战国

青铜

直径 28 厘米，深 16 厘米

Medicine Kettle

Warring States Period

Bronze

Diameter 28 cm/ Depth 16 cm

敞口，折沿，斜腹，一侧有桥形耳，平底，圈足。外部有精美花纹，朱色环带纹上饰黑色菱形纹，其上饰人物运动图，其下画车马人物图，最底部饰朱纹一周。煎药、洗药工具。

北京御生堂中医药博物馆藏

The kettle has a flared mouth, a folded rim, an oblique belly, a flat bottom, a ring-like foot and a bridge-shaped ear on the one side of the belly. The exterior is decorated with the exquisite flower patterns and the red banding is decorated with the black rhombic motifs. The upper part of the banding is decorated with patterns representing the movement of people while the lower part is patterned with the carriage and people. The lowest part of the kettle is decorated with a circle of red pattern. It was used for decocting and washing medicine.

Preserved in Chinese Medicine Museum of Beijing Yu Sheng Tang Drugstore

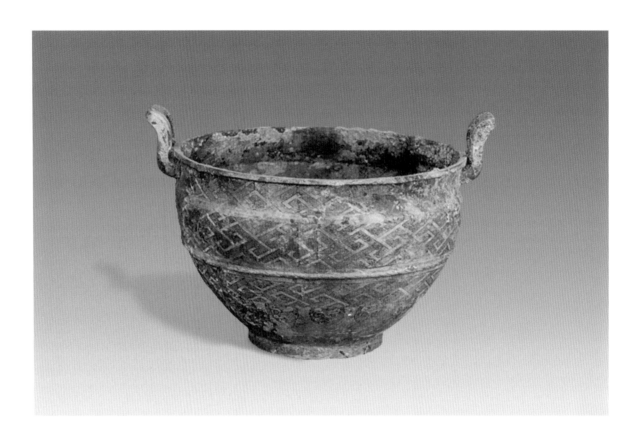

甑

春秋

铜质

口径 33 厘米，通高 25 厘米

Zeng Cauldron

Spring and Autumn Period

Bronze

Mouth Diameter 33 cm/ Height 25 cm

附耳，窄沿，束颈，腹下收，平箅底，附圈足。箅作长条辐射状镂孔。腹饰勾连雷纹、垂叶纹。

山西博物院藏

The cauldron has prick ears, a narrow edge and a contracted neck, a inverted pyramid-like belly, a flat Bi bottom. The pierced Bi is in the shape of radiation. The belly is decorated with thunder pattern and descending leaf pattern.

Preserved in Shanxi Museum

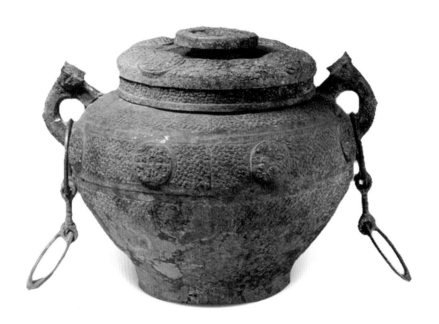

右征君罍

战国

铜质

口径 23.8 厘米，高 37.6 厘米

Lei with Characters "You Zheng Jun"

Warring States Period

Bronze

Mouth Diameter 23.8 cm/ Height 37.6 cm

直口，粗颈，广肩，鼓腹，矮圈足，肩部两兽耳，上覆圆盖圆钮。腹中部凸起一道环带，其上有八个圆涡纹突饰，盖上六个圆涡纹突饰，并饰细密蟠螭纹，带有明显的楚式风格。器口沿上刻有"右征君"三字。

山东博物馆藏

This is a drinking vessel, and it has a straight mouth, a thick neck, a wide shoulder, a swelling belly, a short ring-like foot and a round cover on which there is a round knob. Two beast ears are casted on the shoulder. A streak of ribbon is protruded on the mid belly, on which cut eight circular vertex patterns in relief. There are six protruded circular vertex patterns on the cover which decorated with detailed Pan Chi pattern. The drinking vessel is of clear style of Chu State. "You Zheng Jun" is inscribed on its edge. Preserved in Shandong Museum

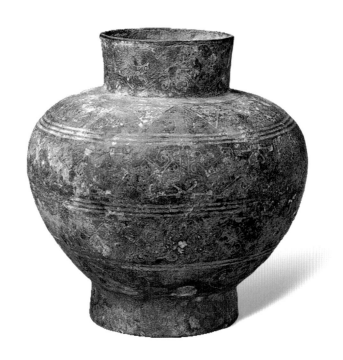

嵌松石缶

战国

铜质

宽 20.6 厘米，通高 19.6 厘米，重 1.78 千克

Fou Inlaid with Turquoise

Warring States Period

Bronze

Width 20.6 cm/ Height 19.6 cm/ Weight 1.78 kg

圆体，直口，硕腹，圈足。器口、腹部饰嵌松石几何纹饰五组，间以弦纹。1981年入藏。

故宫博物院藏

This is a drinking vessel, and it has a round body, a straight mouth, a big belly and a ring-like foot. Five groups of geometrical pattern, which are inlaid with turquoise, are decorated on both the mouth and the belly, with string pattern inscribed among them. The drinking vessel was collected in the year 1981.

Preserved in The Palace Museum

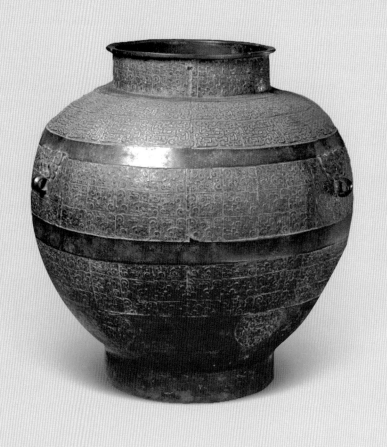

羽纹四耳缶

战国

铜质

口径 21.6 厘米，腹径 42.3 厘米，通高 40 厘米

圆体，直颈，圆肩，大腹，圈足，四兽首衔环耳。颈、腹饰羽状纹，肩饰蟠螭纹，腹下饰垂叶纹，叶内为兽面纹。清宫旧藏。

故宫博物院藏

Four-eared Drinking Vessel Fou Decorated with Feather-like Pattern

Warring States Period

Bronze

Mouth Diameter 21.6 cm/ Belly Diameter 42.3 cm/ Height 40 cm

This Fou wine drinking vessel has a round body, a straight neck, a round shoulders, a big belly, a ring-like foot and four beast-head ears with rings held in their mouth. Feather-like pattern is decorated on both the neck and the belly, while Pan Chi pattern is decorated on the shoulder. Its lower belly is decorated with descending leaf patterns, in which animal mask pattern is decorated. This drinking vessel used to be a collection of the imperial palace of the Qing Dynasty.

Preserved in The Palace Museum

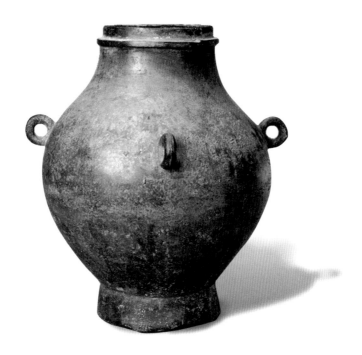

铸客缶

战国后期

铜质

口径 18.4 厘米，宽 46 厘米，通高 46.9 厘米，重 16.22 千克

Fou with Characters "Zhu Ke"

Late Warring States Period

Bronze

Mouth Diameter 18.4 cm/ Width 46 cm/ Height 46.9 cm/ Weight 16.22 kg

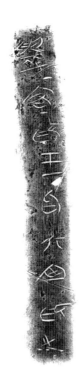

圆体，圈足，大腹，小口，肩部铸有四环，器口外有刻划铭文9字，记外方冶铸匠人"铸客"为王后六室做此缶。1933年安徽寿县朱家集出土，1954年北京市文化局调拨。

故宫博物院藏

This Fou, a drinking vessel, has a round body, a ring-like foot, a big belly, a small mouth and four rings decorated on the shoulders. There is an inscription of 9 characters outside the mouth, recording that "Zhu Ke", the craftsman from outside the region, made this Fou for the imperial harems which belonged to the queen. This drinking vessel was unearthed in Zhujiaji, Shou County, Anhui Province, in 1933 and allocated from Beijing Municipal Bureau of Culture in 1954.

Preserved in The Palace Museum

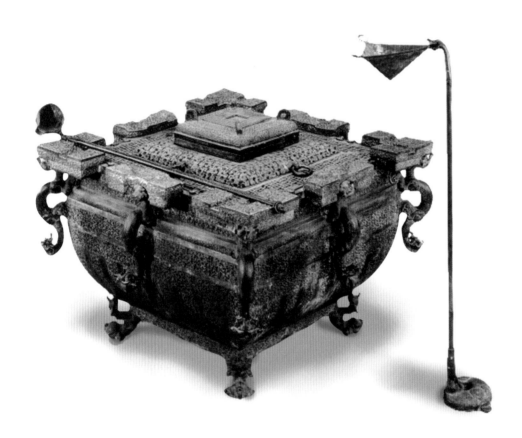

鉴缶及过滤器

战国

铜质

鉴：边长 62 厘米，通高 61.5 厘米

过滤器：杆长 70.8 厘米，通高 88.5 厘米

古代冰（温）酒器。鉴与缶均饰以蟠螭纹、勾连纹和焦叶纹等，均有"曾侯乙作持用终"铭文。鉴圈座附四兽形足，四角，四边共一个攀伏的龙形耳，方形和曲尺形的镂空装饰，方盖面中空，以容纳方尊、缶颈。缶盖呈方形隆起，四角附坚环纽，直口，方唇，溜肩，鼓腹下折内收，圈足，缶身腹部四边各有一坚环耳。1978 年湖北随州擂鼓墩 1 号墓出土。

湖北省博物馆藏

Large Drinking Vessel Jian Fou and the Filter

Warring States Period

Bronze

Vessel: Length 62 cm/ Height 61.5 cm

Filter: Length of the Pole 70.8 cm/ Height 88.5 cm

It was utilized as a wine cooler or wine warmer. The Jian and Fou are decorated with Pan Chi, connected trimming and banana leaf patterns, and both are inscribed with characters, meaning "used by Marquis Yi of Zeng". The Jian, decorated with square hollow-out patterns, has four animal shaped feet and four dragon-shaped ears clawing to each side. The cover is hollowed to accommodate Zun and the neck of Fou. The raised Fou cover with four round knobs on each side has a straight mouth, square lips, sloping shoulders, a swelling belly with its lower region converged and ring-like feet. Four ring-like ears are cast on the belly separately. It was unearthed from No.1 Tomb of Leigudun in Suizhou City, Hubei Province in, 1978.

Preserved in Hubei Provincial Museum

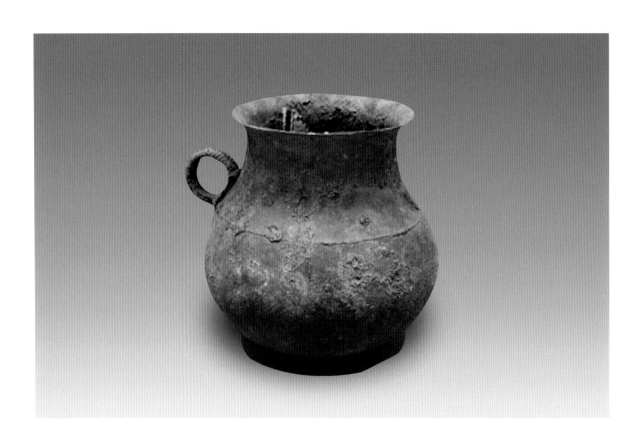

单耳铜鍪

战国

铜质

口径 9 厘米，高 13 厘米

Copper Mou Pot with a Single Ear

Warring States Period

Copper

Mouth Diameter 9 cm/ Height 13 cm

敞口，束颈，腹微鼓，圆底，肩部有一旋纹。
由成都市考古队调拨。

成都中医药大学中医药传统文化博物馆藏

This ancient pot has an open mouth, a
contracted neck, a slightly swelling belly and
a round bottom. A lira pattern is decorated
on the shoulder. It was allocated by Chengdu
Archaeological Team.

Preserved in Museum of Traditional Chinese
Medicine Culture, Chengdu University of
Traditional Chinese Medicine

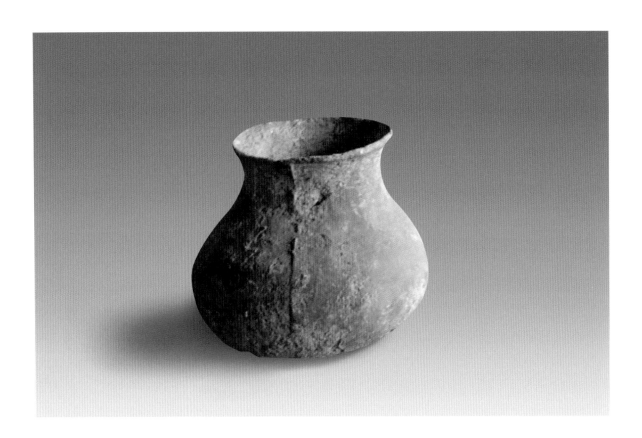

鍪

战国

铜质

口径 9 厘米，高 12 厘米

Ancient Mou Pot

Warring States Period

Copper

Mouth Diameter 9 cm/ Height 12 cm

敞口，束颈，鼓腹，圆底，单耳。炊煮用具。
成都市考古队调拨。

成都中医药大学中医药传统文化博物馆藏

This Mou has an open mouth, a contracted
neck, a swelling belly, a round bottom and
one ear. It was used as cooking utensil. The
ancient pot was allocated by the Chengdu
Archaeological Team.

Preserved in Museum of Traditional Chinese
Medicine Culture, Chengdu University of
Traditional Chinese Medicine

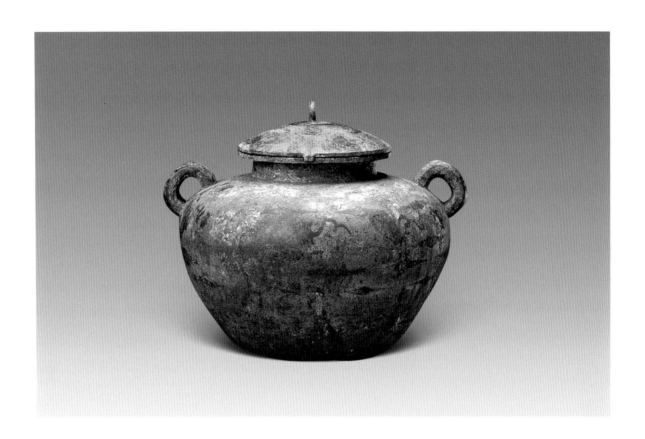

嵌红铜龙纹瓿

战国前期

铜质

宽 44.5 厘米，通高 34.3 厘米，重 10.72 千克

Bu Inlaid with Red Copper Dragon Pattern

Early Warring States Period

Bronze

Width 44.5 cm/ Height 34.3 cm/ Weight 10.72 kg

圆体，大腹，小口，有盖，肩上有二环耳，盖顶部正中有一环。盖、器肩及腹下部饰嵌红铜菱形纹，器腹部饰嵌红铜龙纹。1946 年入藏。

故宫博物院藏

The Bu is a wine container, and it has a round body, a big belly, a small mouth and a cover. There are two rings on the shoulder and one ring in the center of the top of the cover. The lozenge pattern, which is made of inlaid pure copper, is decorated on the cover, shoulder and the lower belly, while dragon pattern made of inlaid pure copper is engraved on the belly. The container was collected in 1946.

Preserved in The Palace Museum

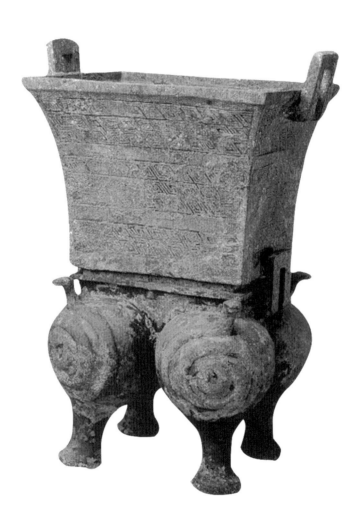

四蛇饰甗

春秋前期

铜质

口径 28.7 厘米×23.2 厘米，宽 33.7 厘米，通高 44.7 厘米，重 12.3 千克

分体式。甑呈长方斗形，直口，附耳，口内无隔，腹高深，上部外侈，下部收敛；平底上有箅孔；甑下有榫圈，是为子口。鬲直口附耳，口内有用来插甑之榫圈的凹形母口；肩四角各饰以盘蛇，上颈昂起，双眼凸于头顶处；腹鼓，似四球相连，分裆线连于腰际；足为蹄形。甑腹饰有三层勾连雷纹，耳饰变体重环纹；鬲腹饰蛇纹，四条盘蛇身上饰鳞纹。1965 年收购。

故宫博物院藏

Yan with Pattern of Four Snakes

Early Spring and Autumn Period

Bronze

Mouth Diameter 28.7 cm×23.2 cm/ Width 33.7 cm/ Height 44.7 cm/ Weight 12.3 kg

The Yan, a cooking vessel, is in a set of two parts. The upper part Zeng is rectangular, flared on the top and convergent at the bottom, with a straight opening, two prick ears decorated with deformed multiple ring-like pattern, a high and deep belly decorated with three layers of thunder pattern. There is a steaming grating on its flat bottom, and a tenon ring under it, called convex smaller mouth. The lower part is Li with prick ears, a straight opening horseshoe feet, and a concave bigger mouth which caves in for inserting the tenon ring of the Zeng. There is a coiling snake with scale pattern on the corners of the shoulder, their neck raised upward and two eyes convex on the head. Its swelling belly with snake pattern looks like conjoint four balls, while its separated-crotch line is connected on the waist. It was collected in 1965.

Preserved in The Palace Museum

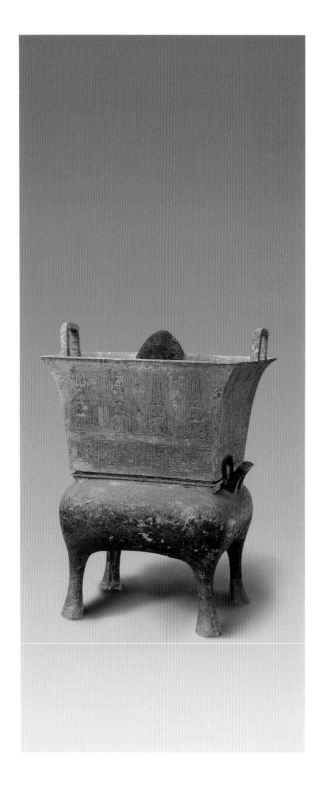

环带纹甗

春秋后期

铜质

宽 47.4 厘米，通高 61.5 厘米，重 28.8 千克

Yan with Wave Pattern

Late Spring and Autumn Period

Bronze

Width 47.4 cm/ Height 61.5 cm/ Weight 28.8 kg

甑为长方深箱形，侈口，立耳，口内有隔。
大腹，腹壁斜收；平底有箅孔；甑下部有
插入鬲口的榫圈。鬲为侈口斜肩，肩上有
一对圆角方耳；平裆，蹄形足。甑体饰环
带纹。1923 年河南新郑出土，1956 年国
家文物局调拨。

故宫博物院藏

The rectangular Zeng utensil has a wide
flared mouth with separation, two side ears, a
big belly with oblique walls and a flat bottom
with holes for steaming grating. Under
the Zeng utensil, there is a tenon ring that
can insert the Zeng utensil into the mouth
of the Li cooking vessel. The Li (cooking
vessel) has a wide flared mouth, an oblique
shoulder on which there is a pair of square
ears with round angle, a flat crotch and
four horseshoe-shaped feet. Wave pattern is
decorated on the Zeng utensil. It was unearthed
in Xinzheng County, Henan Province in 1923
and allocated from State Administration of
Cultural Heritage in 1956.

Preserved in The Palace Museum

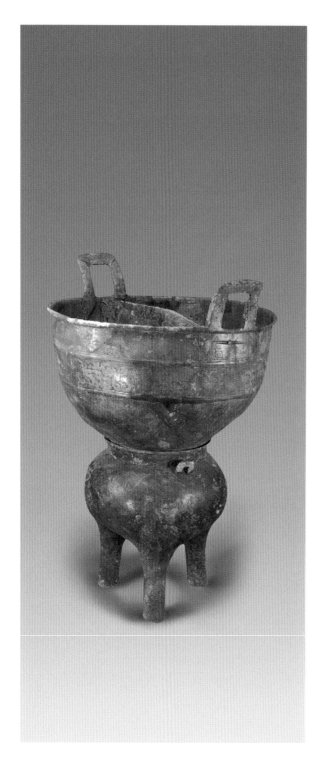

青铜甗

战国初期

铜质

口径 34.8 厘米，通高 58.2 厘米

鬲：口径 20.1 厘米，高 29.1 厘米

Bronze Yan

Early Warring States Period

Bronze

Mouth Diameter 34.8 cm/ Height 58.2 cm

Li: Mouth Diameter 20.1 cm/ Height 29.1 cm

口微敛，方形双耳立于器口，略向外撇。腹外有凸弦纹二道，弦纹之间饰宽体勾连蟠螭纹，弦纹上下饰三角形勾连云雷纹。甑腹内有半圆形铜质活动隔扇装置，可将器内分隔成前后两部分，以便蒸煮不同的两种食品，极为罕见。甑底有长方形箅孔。下部为鬲，有短颈套接甑底，肩部有短小方形双耳，素面无纹。

绍兴市文物管理局藏

The Yan vessel is in a set of two parts. The upper part is Zeng with a slightly contracted mouth and two square upright ears slightly flared outward, two streaks of convex bow-string pattern outside the belly with wide connected Pan Chi pattern in between and connected triangular cloud-thunder pattern on their sides. A moveable semispherical coppery separation-fan separates Zeng into the front and back part for steaming and boiling different kinds of food. On the bottom of Zeng, there are rectangular holes for steaming grating. The lower part is Li, with a short neck that fits with the bottom of Zeng, and two small and short square ears on the shoulder. There is no pattern on Li. Preserved in Shaoxing City Cultural Relics Administration

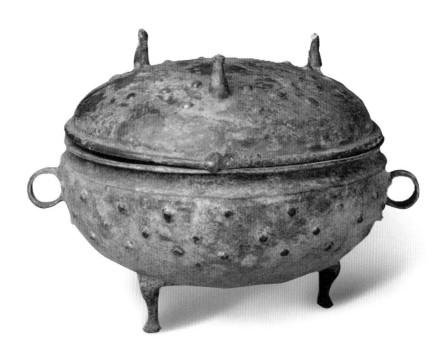

荆公孙敦

春秋后期

铜质

宽 25.2 厘米，通高 17 厘米，重 1.58 千克

Dui with Characters "Jing Gong Sun"

Late Spring and Autumn Period

Bronze

Width 25.2 cm/ Height 17 cm/ Weight 1.58 kg

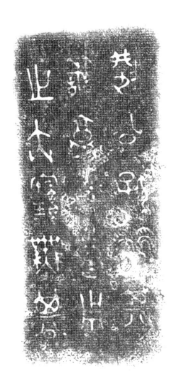

侈口，束颈，耳作环形，圜底下具三个兽蹄足。盖亦有三个蹄形足，可却置。盖、器通饰乳丁纹。盖内有铭文 15 字，记荆公孙自铸食敦，长寿用它，连宝无期。1952 年收购。

故宫博物院藏

The Dui grain receptacle has a wide flared mouth, a contracted neck, two ring-like ears and three beast-shoe-shaped feet. The cover which can serve as another vessel when it is removed from the vessel it covers, also has three beast-shoe-shaped feet. The nipple pattern is decorated on both the cover and the whole body. There is an inscription of 15 characters inside the cover, recording that Jing Gong Sun made this grain receptacle himself, for use for longevity and as a treasure. It was acquired in 1952.

Preserved in The Palace Museum

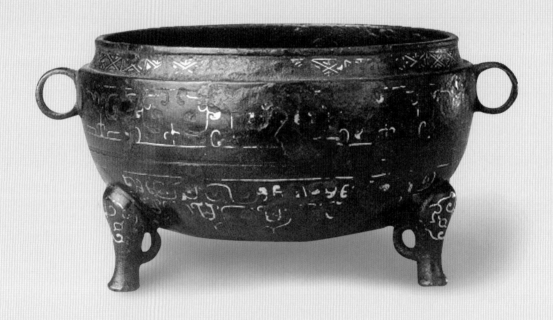

错金云纹敦

战国前期

铜质

口径 16 厘米，宽 21.2 厘米，通高 10.2 厘米，重 1.18 千克

器作半球形，三短足，双环耳。器口沿饰几何纹一周，腹饰流云纹，腹下部饰窃曲纹、垂叶纹，足面饰兽面纹。通体花纹均以错金为饰。清宫旧藏。

故宫博物院藏

Dui with Gold Inlaid Cloud Pattern

Early Spring and Autumn Period

Bronze

Mouth Diameter 16 cm/ Width 21.2 cm/ Height 10.2 cm/ Weight 1.18 kg

The semispherical Dui, a grain receptacle, has three short feet and two ring-like ears. The edge outside the mouth is decorated with geometric pattern, while the belly has flowing cloud pattern and its lower party is decorated with Qie Qu pattern and descending leaf pattern, and the foot surface with animal mask pattern. The patterns of the entire body are inlaid with gold. The grain receptacle was originally a collection of the imperial palace of the Qing Dynasty.

Preserved in The Palace Museum

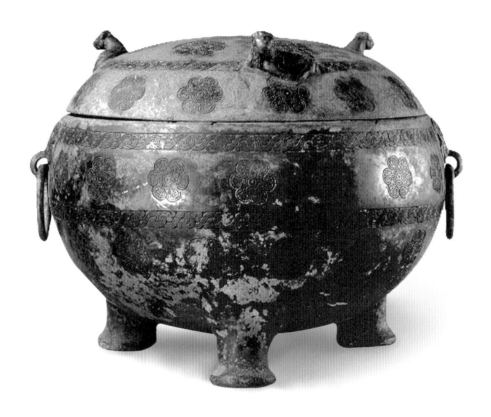

茶花纹敦

战国后期

铜质

宽 24.2 厘米，通高 17.8 厘米，重 3.02 千克

体圆，三短足，双兽首衔环耳，有盖。盖上饰三伏牺，并饰六瓣茶花纹二周，以蟠螭纹一周相隔，器腹上下各饰蟠螭纹一周，中饰六瓣茶花纹。1957 年收购。

故宫博物院藏

Dui with Camellia Pattern

Late Warring States Period

Bronze

Width 24.2 cm/ Height 17.8 cm/ Weight 3.02 kg

This Dui, a grain receptacle, has a round body, three short feet and two ears in the shape of an animal head with rings held in their mouth. It also has a cover, on which there is decoration of three prostrate animals for sacrifice and two streaks of six-petal camellia pattern separated by a round of Pan Chi pattern. Also, there is streak of Pan Chi pattern on the upper and lower belly respectively, with six-petal camellia pattern decorated in the center. It was collected in 1957.

Preserved in The Palace Museum

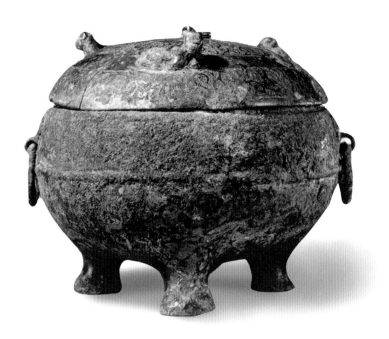

轨敦

战国后期

铜质

口径 19.4 厘米，宽 22.4 厘米，通高 17.8 厘米，重 3.46 千克

Dui with Character "Gui"

Late Warring States Period

Bronze

Mouth Diameter 19.4 cm/ Width 22.4 cm/ Height 17.8 cm/ Weight 3.46 kg

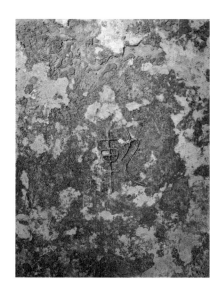

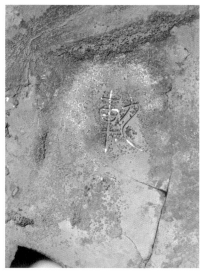

圆体，鼓腹，三短足，双兽面衔环耳，有盖。盖
上饰三伏牺，盖顶有一活环钮，钮下饰相间的叶
状纹与圆涡纹，盖、器各饰枝状纹二周。盖、器
各铸有铭文"轨"字。河南洛阳西宫秦墓出土，
1956 年国家文物局调拨。

故宫博物院藏

This Dui, a grain receptacle, has a round body, a
swelling belly, three short feet, a cover, and two ears
in the shape of an animal mask with rings held in
their mouth. There is a decoration of three prostrate
animals for sacrifice on the cover, and also a
moveable ring-shaped knob on its top, under which
there is decoration of leaf-like pattern alternate with
circular vertex pattern. Both the cover and the body
are decorated with two streaks of branch-like pattern
around them. There is a inscription of a Chinese
character "轨" (Gui) on both the cover and the body
of the vessel. It was unearthed in Qin tomb of West
Palace in Luoyang, Henan Province, and allocated
from State Administration of Cultural Heritage in
1956.

Preserved in The Palace Museum

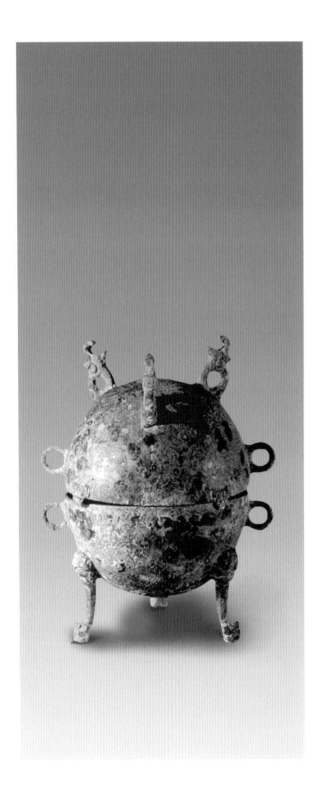

青铜敦

战国后期

铜质

腹径 25.4 厘米，通高 8.8 厘米

Bronze Dui

Late Warring States Period

Bronze

Belly Diameter 25.4 cm/ Height 8.8 cm

其形态，是由鼎和簋相结合演变而成的，呈一个浑圆的球状或椭圆状，由上下两个造型完全相同的三足深腹钵扣合而成，上体为盖，倒置后也可盛食。敦产生于春秋中期，盛行于春秋晚期至战国后期，至秦代已基本消失。此件传世青铜敦是敦在消亡前期的形态的代表作。敦是专门盛黍、稷、稻、粱等粮食作物制成品的盛食具。

上海博物馆藏

Bronze Dui, a grain receptacle in spherical or oval shape, evolved from the combination of a tripod and a Gui (food container), comprised by fastening two bowl-shaped vessels with one on the top and the other the base, both having three feet and a deep belly. The upper part serves as a cover, but when inverted, it serves as a food container. Dui was produced in the mid-Spring and Autumn Period, popular from the late Spring and Autumn Period to the late Warring States Period, and out of use in the Qin Dynasty. It was representative of Dui vessels before its disappearance. Dui was used as food container for broomcorn millet, millet, rice and grain. Preserved in Shanghai Museum

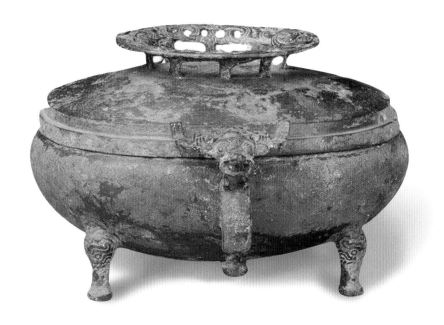

兽耳铒

战国前期

铜质

宽 23.7 厘米，通高 13.8 厘米，重 1.24 千克

He with Animal-shaped Ears

Early Warring States Period

Bronze

Width 23.7 cm/ Height 13.8 cm/ Weight 1.24 kg

椭圆形腹，隆盖，盖顶捉手透空饰有蟠螭纹。腹两侧兽耳作龙形。器腹下侧附有四足，为人面、鸟嘴、双脚、双翼的怪兽。北京市文化局调拨。

故宫博物院藏

This vessel has an oval belly and a raised cover on which the open handle is decorated with Pan Chi pattern. The animal ears are in the shape of a dragon cast on the two sides of the belly. It has four feet under the vessel, which are in the form of an animal with a human face, a beak, two feet and two wings. The vessel was allocated from Beijing Municipal Bureau of Culture.

Preserved in The Palace Museum

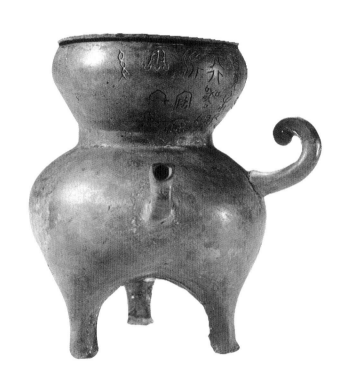

"黄夫人"甗形盉

春秋

铜质

口径 11 厘米，高 18 厘米

"Mrs Huang" Yan-shaped He

Spring and Autumn Period

Bronze

Mouth Diameter 11 cm/ Height 18 cm

敛口尖唇，平盖，卷尾鋬，兽头流，器内
有一圆形无孔箅。口沿下铸有铭文："黄
子作黄甫（夫）人行器，则永宝宝霝冬（终）
霝复"。1983 年河南省光山宝相寺黄君
孟夫妇合葬墓出土。

河南博物院藏

This is a vessel for holding water or wine,
and it has a contracted mouth with sharp rim,
a flat cover, a handle shaped like a coiling
tail, a beast-head spout, and there is a round
grate without holes. There is an inscription
below the mouth's edge on the outside
meaning that this Yan-shaped vessel was
made by the Head of the Huang Kingdom in
early Spring and Autumn Period for his wife.
It was unearthed in a joint burial tomb of the
Head of Huang Kingdom named Meng and
his wife in Baoxiang Temple, Guangshan,
Henan Province, in 1983.

Preserved in Henan Museum

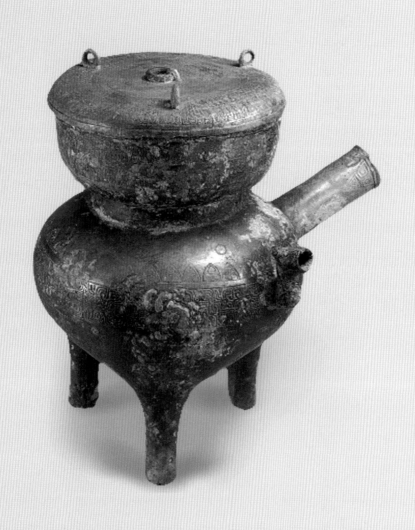

青铜盉

战国初期

铜质

高 26 厘米

上部为带盖甑，下部为鬲式带把盉，甑体明显小于杯体。

浙江省博物馆藏

Bronze He

Early Warring States Period

Bronze

Height 26 cm

This vessel consists of two parts. The upper part of this vessel is a "Zeng" with a cover, a cooking vessel structure, while the lower part is a He with a handle, shaped like a Li, a cooking vessel. The upper part is obviously smaller than the lower part.

Preserved in Zhejiang Provincial Museum

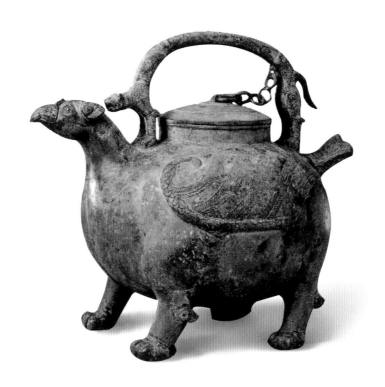

鸟形盉

战国前期

铜质

宽 30.4 厘米，通高 26.3 厘米，重 3.39 千克

Bird-shaped He

Early Warring States Period

Bronze

Width 30.4 cm/ Height 26.3 cm/ Weight 3.39 kg

器整体作立鸟形，虎形提梁，四兽足，鸟
首上喙与鼻间以活环相连，倒水时可自动
张开。翼饰大尾凤纹，足、流尾均为分铸
后与器身拼合为一体。1946 年入藏。

故宫博物院藏

This is a drinking vessel, shaped like a
standing bird. It has a tiger-shaped loop
handle and four animal hoof-like feet.
The upper beak is linked with the nose
by movable rings, which will open when
pouring water. There is phoenix pattern
with a big tail on the wings. Its feet and the
flow tail were cast separately, and were put
together with the body. This bird-shaped
drinking vessel was collected in 1946.
Preserved in The Palace Museum

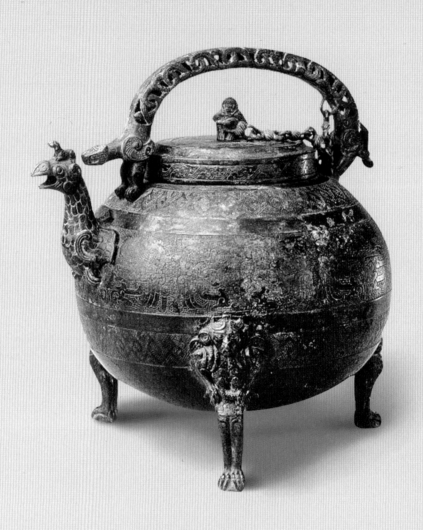

螭梁盉

战国前期

铜质

宽 24.2 厘米，通高 24.2 厘米，重 3.52 千克

圆体，直口，硕腹，三人形足，鸟首形流，提梁为一蟠螭形，有盖，平顶，正中为一猴形纽，梁与盖纽间以挂链相连。器腹饰蟠螭纹及粟纹，盖口饰蟠虺纹，盖顶饰云纹。清宫旧藏。

故宫博物院藏

He with a Handle Shaped Like a Hornless Dragon

Early Warring States Period

Bronze

Width 24.2 cm/ Height 24.2 cm/ Weight 3.52 kg

This vessel has a round body, a straight mouth, a big belly, three human-shaped feet, a bird head-shaped spout, and a loop handle shaped like a hornless dragon, a flat cover with a monkey-shaped knob on its center. The loop handle is linked to the knob by a chain. The belly of the vessel is decorated with Pan Chi pattern and millet-like pattern, while the mouth of the cover is decorated with Pan Hui pattern. There is cloud pattern on the top of the cover. It was originally an article in the imperial palace of the Qing Dynasty.

Preserved in The Palace Museum

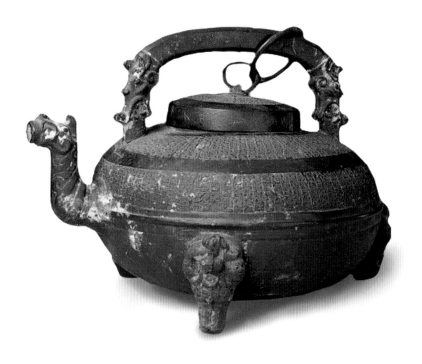

铸客盉

战国后期

铜质

宽 32.5 厘米，通高 21.9 厘米，重 3.52 千克

He with Characters "Zhu Ke"

Late Warring States Period

Bronze

Width 32.5 cm/ Height 21.9 cm/ Weight 3.52 kg

圆体，鼓腹，有流，流作兽首形，三铁铸短足，有梁，有盖，梁两端饰兽首，梁与盖间以二环相连。盖、腹上部饰细羽状纹。盖外侧、器口旁各有刻划对铭1行7字，记外方冶铸匠人"铸客"为供王之饮食酒馔的机构做此盉。1933年安徽寿县朱家集出土，1957年北京市文化局调拨。

故宫博物院藏

This is a drinking vessel, and it has a round body, a swelling belly, an animal head-shaped spout, three short feet cast with iron, a loop handle and a cover. Both ends of the loop handle are decorated with animal head, and the handle is linked to the cover by two rings. The cover and the upper part of the belly are decorated with fine feather-like pattern. There is a one-line inscription of 7 characters respectively outside the cover and on the surface next to the mouth, recording that "Zhu Ke", a craftsman from outside the region, cast this drinking vessel for the institution supplying food and drinking for the king. It was unearthed in Zhujiaji, Shouxian County, Anhui Province, in 1933, and was allocated from Beijing Municipal Bureau of Culture in 1957. Preserved in The Palace Museum

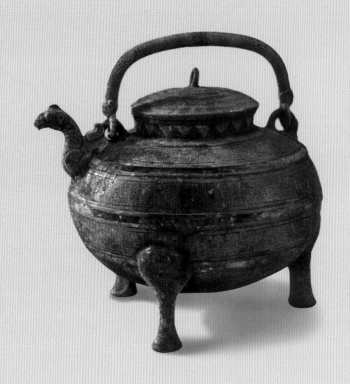

蟠虺纹铜盉

战国

铜质

腹径 21 厘米，通高 20.4 厘米

Bronze He with Pan Hui Pattern

Warring States Period

Bronze

Belly Diameter 21 cm/ Height 20.4 cm

此盉虽出土于西汉墓中，但其平唇、短颈、广肩、扁圆腹的造型，以及器身上三圈蟠虺纹饰的纹样特征，都透露出浓厚的战国青铜器的气息。尤其是那喙口微张的凤鸟形短流，写实意味很浓，与西汉时期流行的可以自由开合鸟形流上喙的做法迥然有别，却与西周至春秋战国青铜盉上流口大小固定不变的风格相吻合。1991年邗江甘泉巴家墩西汉木椁墓出土。

扬州博物馆藏

This vessel was unearthed from the tomb of the western Han Dynasty, and has a flat rim, a short neck, a wide shoulders, a flattened round belly and three circles of Pan Hui pattern around the body, especially the phoenix-shaped spout with a slightly opened beak reflecting a strong sense of realism, and differing from the moveable beak of bird-shaped spout popular in the Western Han Dynasty, but matches the style from the Western Zhou Dynasty to the Spring and Autumn and Warring States Period. It was unearthed in Western Han Dynasty Muchun Tomb, Ganquan, Hanjiang, in 1991.

Preserved in Yangzhou Museum

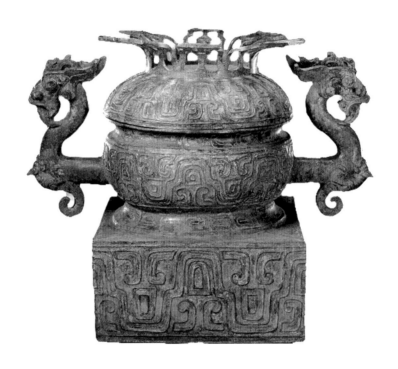

龙耳簋

春秋后期

铜质

口径 23.1 厘米，宽 43 厘米，通高 33.9 厘米，重 11.45 千克

Gui with Dragon-shaped Ears

Late Spring and Autumn Period

Bronze

Mouth Diameter 23.1 cm/ Width 43 cm/ Height 33.9 cm/ Weight 11.45 kg

侈口，束颈，双龙耳，矮体宽腹，圈足下
连方座。盖捉手作莲瓣状，中央饰蟠虺纹；
盖边、腹、方座饰云带纹并间以重环纹。
1959 年收购。

故宫博物院藏

This is a food container, and it has a wide
flared mouth, a contracted neck, two dragon-
shaped ears, a short body, a wide belly and a
ring-like foot connected with a square pedestal
below. The knob of the cover is in the shape of
lotus petal with Pan Hui pattern in the center.
The cloud ribbon-like pattern alternate with
multiple ring-like pattern decorates the edge of
the cover, the belly, and the square pedestal.
It was acquired in 1959.
Preserved in The Palace Museum

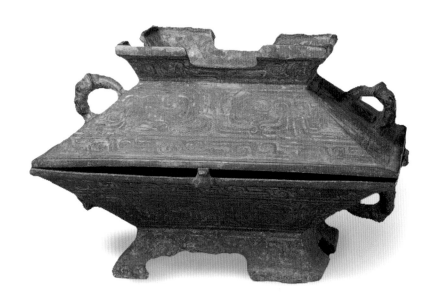

铸子叔黑𦣞簠

春秋前期

铜质

宽 27.6 厘米，通高 17.8 厘米，重 4.24 千克

Fu with Characters Includes "Shu Hei"

Early Spring and Autumn Period

Bronze

Width 27.6 cm/ Height 17.8 cm/ Weight 4.24 kg

器壁斜，腹较浅，有简化的兽首形环耳，方圈足的底边均有"冂"形缺口。盖可却置。器、盖对铭各 4 行 17 字。传光绪初年出土于山东桓台，1964 年收购。

故宫博物院藏

This is a square grain receptacle that has oblique walls, a slightly shallow belly, simplified animal head-shaped ears and a square ring-like foot with a "冂"shape breach on its bottom edge. The cover can serve as another vessel when it is removed from the vessel it covers. A 4–line inscription of 17 characters is on both the body and the cover. It is said that this square grain receptacle was unearthed in Huantai, Shandong Province, in the early period of the reign of Guangxu Emperor, the 11th emperor of the Qing Dynasty, and was collected in 1964.

Preserved in The Palace Museum

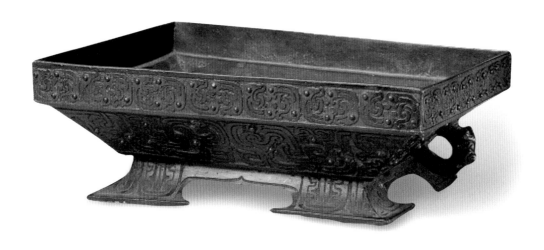

叔朕簠

春秋后期

铜质

宽 30 厘米，通高 10.3 厘米，重 3.72 千克

Fu with Characters "Shu Zhen"

Late Spring and Autumn Period

Bronze

Width 30 cm/ Height 10.3 cm/ Weight 3.72 kg

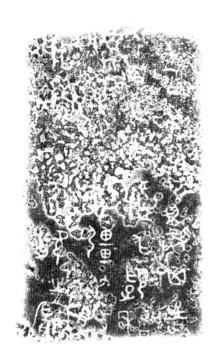

长方形，直口，折壁，腹较深，方圈足的各边有缺。折壁上有兽头环耳。器身饰蟠螭纹。器内有 5 行 37 字铭文。国家文物局调拨。

故宫博物院藏

This rectangular grain receptacle has a straight mouth, folded walls, a deep belly and a square ring-like foot with a breach on each side. Animal-head ring ears are cast on the folded wall, while Pan Chi pattern is decorated on the body. Inside the receptacle, there is a inscription of 37 characters in 5 lines meaning "it was made for praying for a good harvest and longevity". It was allocated from State Administration of Cultural Heritage. Preserved in The Palace Museum

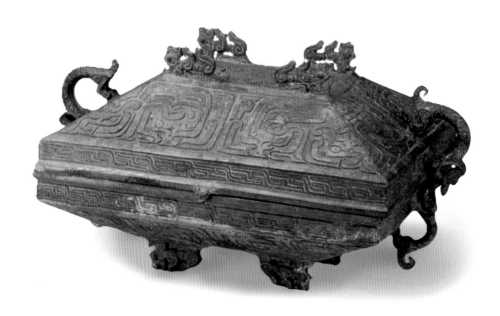

兽纹铜簠

春秋

铜质

高 17.5 厘米

Copper Fu with Animal Patterns

Spring and Autumn Period

Copper

Height 17.5 cm

长方形器，盖与底完全相同，子母口，盖沿附小兽头，使其扣合牢固。上腹垂直，下腹斜向内收，长方形平底，四足为疾走的小兽，两耳作长髯卷尾的小兽，拱背蹲足。口沿下饰窃曲纹，腹下部饰象首纹，盖与底纹饰相同。

山东博物馆藏

This vessel is rectangular with a cover that matches the bottom in size and a snap-lid. Two small animal head-shaped decorations attached along the cover edge help fasten the grain receptacle. Its upper part of the belly is vertical, while its lower part is oblique inwards. This vessel has a flat bottom, four small feet in the shape of trotty animals, and two ears are in the shape of small animals with long whiskers, curved tails, hogback and squat feet. There is Qie Qu pattern below the edge of the mouth, elephant-head pattern on the lower part of the belly. The cover and the bottom have the same pattern.

Preserved in Shandong Museum

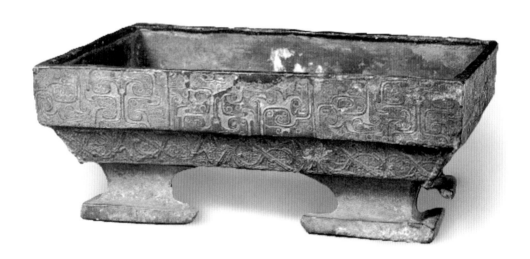

楚王酓朏簠

战国后期

铜质

长 31.8 厘米，宽 21.7 厘米，通高 11.7 厘米，重 5.08 千克

Fu with Characters "Chu Wang Yan Fei"

Late Spring and Autumn Period

Bronze

Length 31.8 cm/ Width 21.7 cm/ Height 11.7 cm/ Weight 5.08 kg

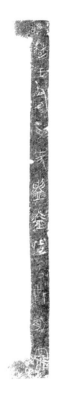

长方形，方足中空。腹饰云纹。器口有刻划铭文14字。1959年北京市文化局调拨。

故宫博物院藏

The rectangular Fu is a grain receptacle, and it has hollow square feet. The cloud pattern decorates its belly. There is an inscription of 14 characters on the mouth. It was allocated from Beijing Municipal Bureau of Culture in 1959.

Preserved in The Palace Museum

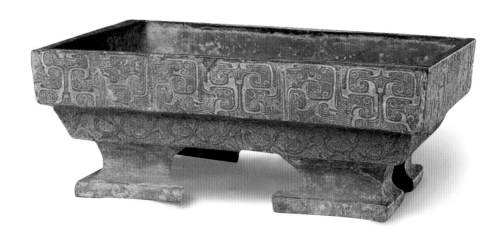

楚王酓朏簠

战国后期

铜质

长 32.4 厘米，宽 21.6 厘米，通高 11.8 厘米，重 5.26 千克

Fu with Characters "Chu Wang Yan Fei"

Late Warring States Period

Bronze

Length 32.4 cm/ Width 21.6 cm/ Height 11.8 cm/ Weight 5.26 kg

长方形，方足中空。腹饰云纹。器口有刻划铭文 12 字，记楚王酓朏做此金簠，以供每岁尝祭祀之用。1959 年北京市文化局调拨。

故宫博物院藏

This rectangular Fu is a grain receptacle, and it has hollow square feet. The cloud pattern decorates on the belly. There is an inscription of 12 characters on the mouth, recording that Yan Fei, king of Chu Kingdom, made this gold grain receptacle for the annual sacrifice. It was allocated from Beijing Municipal Bureau of Culture in 1959.

Preserved in The Palace Museum

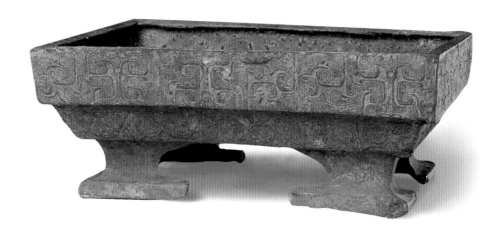

楚王禽脂簠

战国后期

铜质

长 31.9 厘米，宽 21.7 厘米，通高 12 厘米，重 5 千克

Fu with Characters "Chu Wang Yan Fei"

Late Warring States Period

Bronze

Length 31.9 cm/ Width 21.7 cm/ Height 12 cm/ Weight 5 kg

长方形，方足中空。腹饰云纹。器口上有
刻划铭文 12 字，记楚王酓朏铸此金簠，
以供每岁尝祭之用。1959 年北京市文化
局调拨。

故宫博物院藏

The rectangular Fu is a grain receptacle, and
it has hollow square feet. The cloud pattern
decorates the belly. There is an inscription
of 12 characters on the mouth, recording
that Yan Fei, king of Chu Kingdom, made
this grain receptacle for the annual sacrifice.
It was allocated from Beijing Municipal
Bureau of Culture in 1959.

Preserved in The Palace Museum

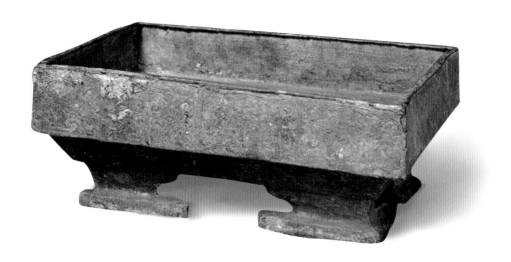

铸客簠

战国后期

铜质

长 31.6 厘米，宽 21.7 厘米，通高 12.5 厘米，重 2.18 千克

Fu with Characters "Zhu Ke"

Late Warring States Period

Bronze

Length 31.6 cm/ Width 21.7 cm/ Height 12.5 cm/ Weight 2.18 kg

长方形，四方足，腹饰由云雷纹组成的几
何纹。器口有刻划铭文9字，记外方冶铸
匠人"铸客"为王后六室做此簠。1933
年安徽寿县朱家集出土，1959 年北京市
文化局调拨。

故宫博物院藏

The rectangular Fu is a grain receptacle,
and it has four square feet, a belly with
geometrical pattern composed of cloud-
thunder pattern. There is an inscription of
9 characters along the edge of the mouth,
recording that "Zhu Ke", the craftsman from
outside the region, made this "He" for the
imperial harems which belongs to the queen.
It was unearthed in Zhujiaji, Shouxian
County, Anhui Province, in 1933. It was
allocated from Beijing Municipal Bureau of
Culture in 1959.

Preserved in The Palace Museum

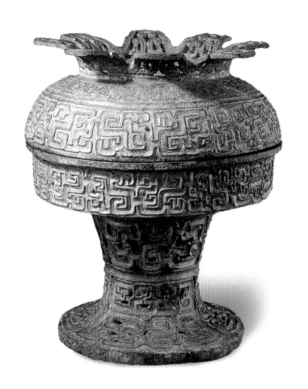

鲁大司徒簠

春秋后期

铜质

宽 25.2 厘米，通高 28.6 厘米，重 7.24 千克

Fu with Characters "Lu Da Si Tu"

Late Spring and Autumn Period

Bronze

Width 25.2 cm/ Height 28.6 cm/ Weight 7.24 kg

直口，浅盘，平底，圈足，腰部有一束箍。盖上有花瓣形捉手，可却置。整器饰以变体的蟠虺纹，盖的捉手和圈足镂空。盖、器对铭，各4行25字，记鲁国的大司徒厚氏元自做盛食的器皿。1932年山东曲阜林前村出土，1961年国家文物局调拨。

故宫博物院藏

Fu is a type of food container, and it has a straight mouth, a shallow plate, a flat bottom and a ring-like foot. A hank of hoop decorates the waist. The cover, which can serve as another vessel when it is removed from the vessel it covers, has a petal-shaped handle. The entire body is decorated with deformative Pan Hui pattern, while the handle of the cover and the ring-like foot are hollow. There is a inscription of 25 characters in 4 lines both on the cover and the body. It was unearthed in Linqian Village, Qufu, Shandong Province in 1932, and allocated from State Administration of Cultural Heritage in 1961.

Preserved in The Palace Museum   .

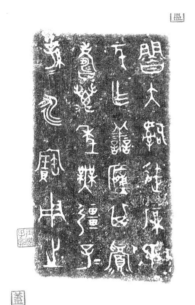

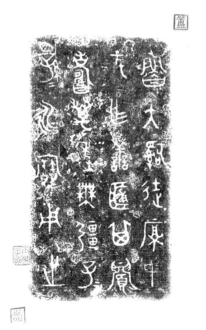

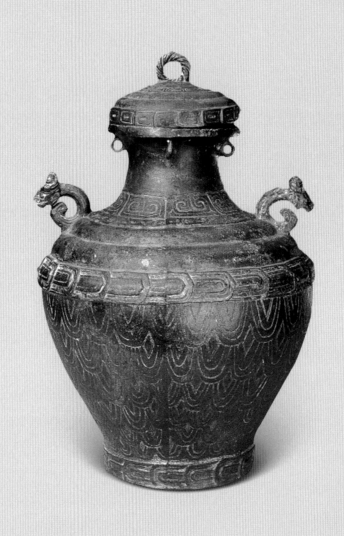

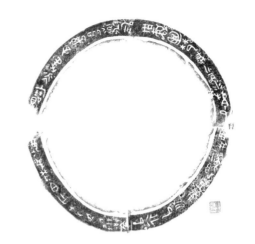

郑义伯醽

春秋前期

铜质

口径 14.7 厘米，通高 45.5 厘米，重 9.66 千克

侈口，细颈，硕腹，附兽耳。有盖，盖口纳于颈中。盖纽如绳，盖顶及边均饰一道重环纹，器口下饰回纹，颈饰窃曲纹，腹饰鳞纹，鳞纹上、下又各饰一道相向的瓦纹。盖、器铭文大意相同，盖口外壁有 8 行 33 字；器颈部有 32 字，呈环行排列。清宫旧物（原藏颐和园）。

故宫博物院藏

Ling with Characters "Zheng Yi Bo"

Early Spring and Autumn Period

Bronze

Mouth Diameter 14.7 cm/ Height 45.5 cm/ Weight 9.66 kg

Ling is a type of container for holding water, and it has a wide flared mouth, a thin neck, a big belly and two animal-shaped ears. It has a cover, whose opening fits into the neck, and the knob in rope-like. A streak of multiple ring-like pattern decorates both the cover's top and the edges, and rectangular spiral pattern decorates the area below the mouth of the vessel on the outside. Its neck is decorated with Qie Qu pattern, and the belly with scale-like pattern, and above and under the pattern there is a streak of tile-like pattern respectively. There's an inscription of 33 characters in 8 lines on the outside wall of the mouth of the cover, while an inscription of 32 characters is arranged in a ring form on the neck. It was originally a collection of the imperial palace of the Qing Dynasty (originally collected by the Summer Palace).

Preserved in The Palace Museum

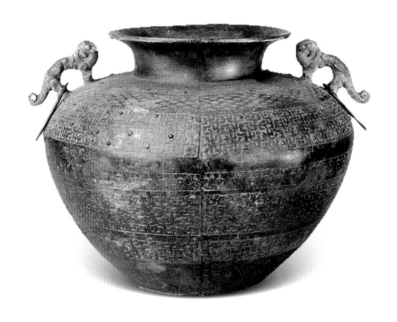

蟠虺纹罍

春秋后期

铜质

口径 24.6 厘米，通高 32.5 厘米，重 7.08 千克

Ling with Pan Hui Pattern

Late Spring and Autumn Period

Bronze

Mouth Diameter 24.6 cm/ Height 32.5 cm/ Weight 7.08 kg

大口外侈，有一周平边；颈大而短；广肩，
上饰双兽耳，耳上套环；大腹，平底。以
蟠虺纹为主题纹饰。清宫旧物（原藏颐和
园）。

故宫博物院藏

Ling is a drinking vessel serving for holding
water, and it has a wide flared mouth with
a flat edge, a thick and short neck, wide
shoulders with two animal-shaped ears with
a ring, a big belly and a flat bottom. Pan Hui
pattern is used as the major pattern on this
drinking vessel. It was originally preserved
in the imperial palace of the Qing Dynasty
(originally collected by the Summer Palace).
Preserved in The Palace Museum

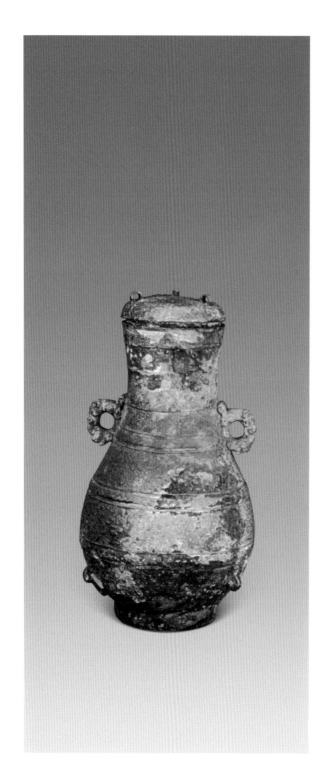

蟠虺纹盖壶

春秋

铜质

口径 11.1 厘米，腹径 20.4 厘米，通高 34 厘米

Pot with a Cover with Pan Hui Pattern

Spring and Autumn Period

Bronze

Mouth Diameter 11.1 cm/ Belly Diameter 20.4 cm/

Height 34 cm

隆盖，三环纽。子口微敞，高束颈，溜肩，鼓腹下收，矮圈足。颈饰螭纹环耳一对，下腹部饰三纽衔环。盖面饰雷纹地卷云纹，口外凸饰蟠螭纹宽带一周。

山西博物院藏

This pot has a raised cover, three ring-like knobs, a slightly flared mouth, a high contracted neck, a sloping shoulders, a swelling belly with its lower region converged, and a short ring-like foot. A pair of ring-like ears are decorated with Chi pattern casted on the neck, while three knobs, which hold rings, are decorated on the lower belly. The thunder and cloud pattern is engraved on the surface of the cover, while a round of wide ribbon of protruded Pan Chi pattern is decorated outside the mouth.
Preserved in Shanxi Museum

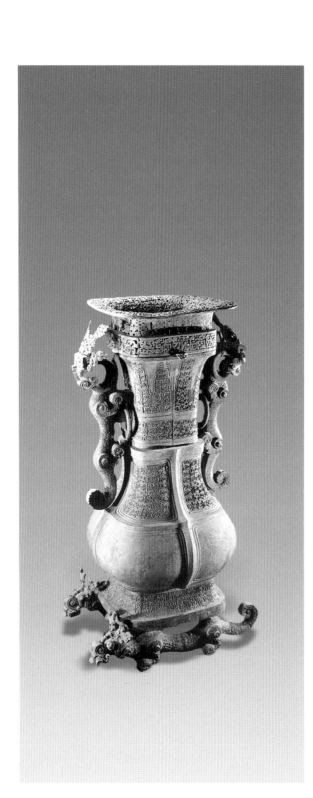

龙耳方壶

春秋

铜质

通高 79.2 厘米

口：长 22.7 厘米，宽 18.8 厘米

Square Pot with Dragon Ears

Spring and Autumn Period

Bronze

Height 79.2 cm

Mouth: Length 22.7 cm/ Width 18.8 cm

侈口，细长颈，龙形双耳，垂腹，方圈足，虎形器座。口上有中空冠盖，四壁镂空成蟠虺纹。器身饰蕉叶纹，腹部四壁起脊，上部饰有变形蟠虺纹，下部素面。1978年河南省淅川下寺1号楚墓出土。

河南博物院藏

The pot has a flared mouth, a thin and long neck, two dragon-like ears, a vertical belly, a square ring-like foot and a tiger-shaped pedestal. There is a hollow crown cover on the mouth, of which four walls are engraved into hollow Pan Hui pattern. Banana leaf pattern is decorated on its body, with ridges casted on four walls of the belly. The upper belly is decorated with deformative Pan Hui pattern, while no pattern is engraved on the lower belly. The square pot was unearthed in the No.1 Chu tombs in Xiasi Village, Xichuan County, Henan Province, in 1978. Preserved in Henan Museum

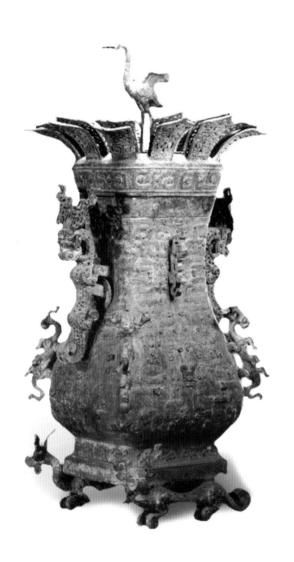

莲鹤方壶

春秋

铜质

口径 31 厘米，高 120 厘米

Square Pot with Patterns of Lotus Petal and Cranes

Spring and Autumn Period

Bronze

Mouth Diameter 31 cm/ Height 120 cm

长方形口，上有盖，长颈，龙形双耳，垂腹，圈足。盖上饰两层盛开莲瓣，中立一鹤。腹部满饰龙纹，四角各攀附有一立体小兽。圈足下有两只怪兽，以背承器。1923 年河南省新郑市城关乡李家楼出土。

河南博物院藏

The pot has a rectangular mouth, a long neck, two dragon-like ears, a vertical belly and a ring-like foot. Two layers of blooming petals are decorated on the cover, with a crane standing in the center. The whole belly is engraved with dragon pattern, with a little solid beast respectively attached on four angles. Under the pot, there are two monsters holding the pot with their back. It was unearthed in Lijialou, Chengguan Township, Xinzheng City, Henan Province, in 1923. Preserved in Henan Museum

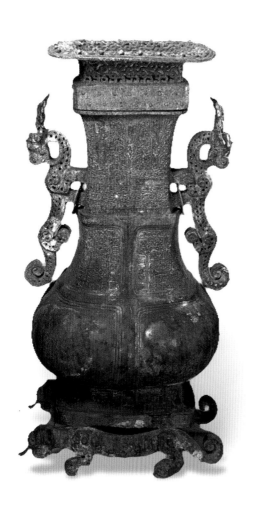

兽耳虎足方壶

春秋后期

铜质

宽 47.2 厘米，通高 87.5 厘米，重 41 千克

Square Pot with Animal Ears and Tiger Feet

Late Spring and Autumn Period

Bronze

Width 47.2 cm/ Height 87.5 cm/ Weight 41 kg

体椭方，长颈，鼓腹，有盖。盖铸透空的蟠虺纹；颈饰蕉叶纹；双龙耳上铸有细镂孔；腹饰界栏状凸棱，上区饰蟠虺纹；圈足饰蟠虺纹和云纹，下卧二虎。1923年河南新郑出土，1956年国家文物局调拨。

故宫博物院藏

The pot has an oval and square body, a long neck, a swelling belly and a cover. Hollow Pan Hui pattern is decorated on the cover, while banana leaf pattern is engraved on the neck. On the two dragon ears, there are thin hollow holes, while protruded fence-like ridge is decorated on the belly, with Pan Hui pattern carved on the upper region. The ring-like foot is decorated with Pan Hui pattern and cloud pattern, under which are engraved two lying tigers. The pot was unearthed in Xinzheng, Henan Province, in 1923. It was allocated from State Administration of Cultural Heritage in 1956.

Preserved in The Palace Museum

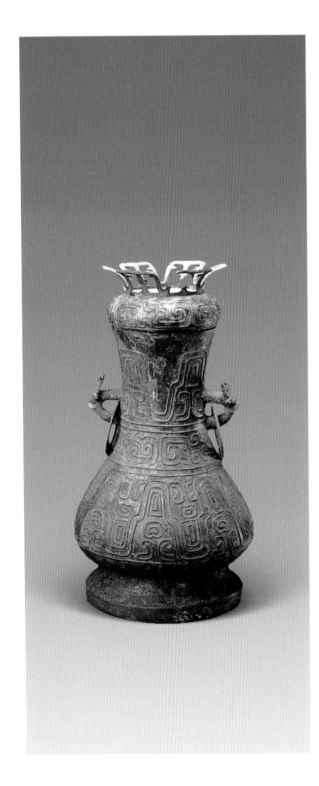

环带纹壶

春秋后期

铜质

宽 25 厘米，通高 43.5 厘米，重 8.11 千克

Pot with Ribbon-like Pattern

Late Spring and Autumn Period

Bronze

Width 25 cm/ Height 43.5 cm/ Weight 8.11 kg

长颈，侈口，腹较圆，颈部有兽首衔环耳。盖冠镂孔作花瓣状。盖沿及颈的下部饰窃曲纹，器腹、圈足和颈上部饰有不同形态的环带纹。1923 年河南新郑出土，1959 年北京市文化局调拨。

故宫博物院藏

The pot has a long neck, a flared mouth and a round belly. On the neck, there are two beast-head ears with rings held in the mouth. The top of the cover is hollowed out to form the petals of a flower and Qie Qu pattern decorates the edge and the lower neck, while different forms of ribbon-like patterns are engraved on the belly, ring-like foot and the upper neck. It was unearthed in Xinzheng, Henan Province, in 1923 and allocated from Beijing Municipal Bureau of Culture, in 1959.

Preserved in The Palace Museum

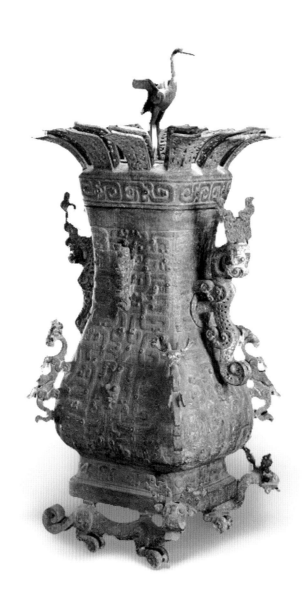

立鹤方壶

春秋后期

铜质

宽 54 厘米，通高 122 厘米，重 64 千克

方壶，形体巨大。全器布局对称。透空的双龙耳较大，上出器口，下及器腹；壶体四面以蟠龙纹为主体纹饰，并在腹部四角各铸一飞龙；圈足下以两只伏虎承器。双层透空莲瓣上立有一只展翅欲飞、引颈高歌的仙鹤。1923 年河南新郑出土，1956 年国家文物局调拨。

故宫博物院藏

Square Pot with Standing Crane

Late Spring and Autumn Period

Bronze

Width 54 cm/ Height 122 cm/ Weight 64 kg

This rectangular pot has a huge body, and is symmetrical in layout. Two big hollowed-out dragon-shaped ears on flanks of the pot are higher than the mouth, and a flying dragon is cast on each corner of its belly. Four sides of the body are mainly decorated with patterns of coiled dragon. Two lying tigers lie under the ring-like foot to support the vessel. On its cover decorations of two layers of openwork lotus petals stands a fluttering and singing crane. This pot was unearthed in Xinzheng of Henan Province in 1923 and allocated from State Administration of Cultural Heritage in 1956.

Preserved in The Palace Museum

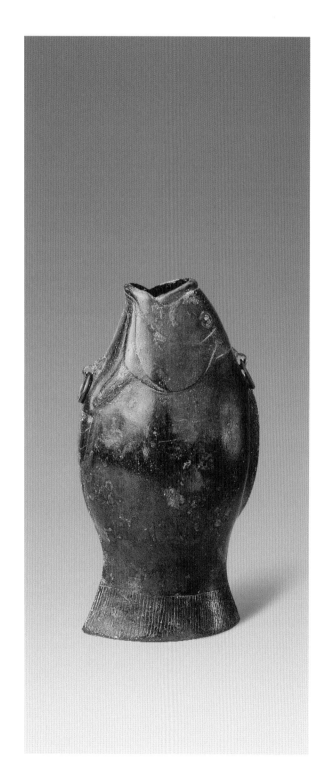

鱼形壶

战国前期

铜质

宽 18 厘米，足径 15.5 厘米，通高 32.5 厘米，

重 2.4 千克

Fish-shaped Pot

Early Warring States Period

Bronze

Width 18 cm/ Foot Diameter 15.5 cm/ Height 32.5 cm/

Weight 2.4 kg

通体作立鱼形，鱼口向上，鱼尾向下为足，鱼腹、背上部有兽首衔环，鱼眼嵌金为饰。清宫旧藏。

故宫博物院藏

The whole body of this pot is made in the shape of fish. The mouth of the fish is upwards, and the foot is shaped like a fish tail. There is an animal head-shaped ear with rings held in the mouth both on the belly and back of the fish. The eyes of fish are inlaid with gold as decorations. The vessel used to be a collection of the imperial palace of the Qing Dynasty. Preserved in The Palace Museum

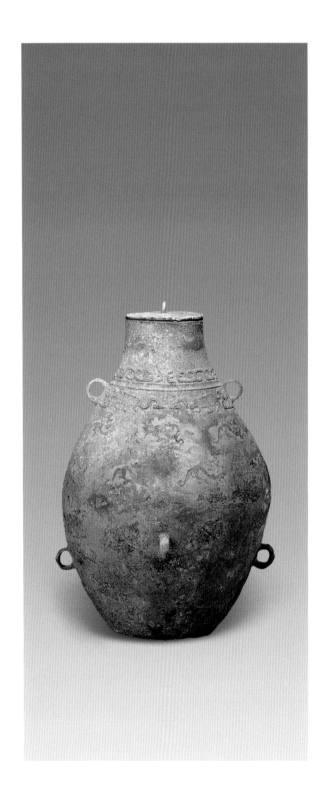

嵌赤铜象纹五环带盖壶

战国前期

铜质

宽 37 厘米，通高 52 厘米，重 7.34 千克

Pot with Red Copper-inlaid Elephant Pattern

Early Warring States Period

Bronze

Width 37 cm/ Height 52 cm/ Weight 7.34 kg

体扁圆，附铸环五，有盖，盖上饰三嵌铜
兽纹，正中一环。器颈饰勾连边纹，肩饰
四象纹，腹饰嵌铜兽纹三周。1959年入藏。

故宫博物院藏

The flattened circular body has five rings cast
around it. The cover is decorated with three
inlaid copper-animal patterns, and there is a
ring in the center of the cover. The neck is
decorated with connected trimming patterns.
The shoulder is decorated with four elephant
patterns. The belly is decorated with 3 circles
of copper-inlaid animal patterns. It was
collected in 1959.

Preserved in The Palace Museum

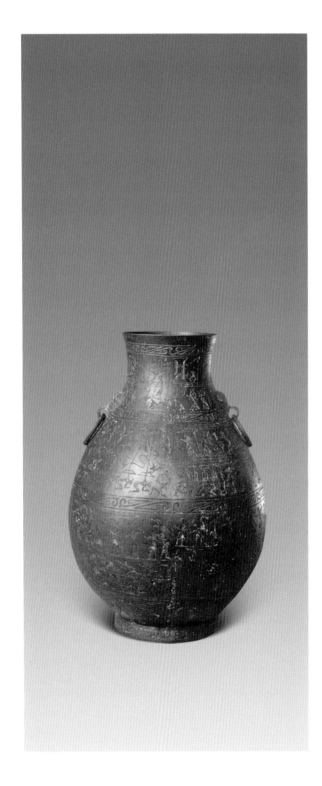

宴乐渔猎攻战纹图壶

战国前期

铜质

口径 10.9 厘米，宽 22.3 厘米，足径 11.9 厘米，

通高 31.6 厘米，重 3.54 千克

Pot with Patterns of Feasting, Fishing, Hunting and Fighting Scenes

Early Warring States Period

Bronze

Mouth Diameter 10.9 cm/ Width 22.3 cm/ Foot Diameter 11.9 cm/ Height 31.6 cm/ Weight 3.54 kg

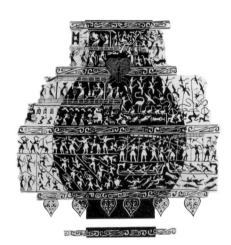

圆体，侈口，双兽首衔环，圈足。器身被四圈三角云雷纹分为三层，其间分别饰编钟乐舞、宴乐、狩猎，以及水陆攻战纹饰，足上方饰蕉叶纹一周，圈足饰三角云雷纹。铸造工艺精良，纹饰图案生动。1946 年入藏。

故宫博物院藏

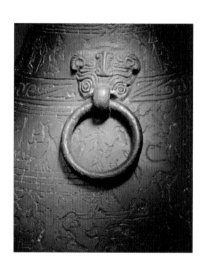

The round body of this vessel has a flared mouth, two ring-shaped handles hanging down from beast heads and a ring-like foot. The body is divided into three sections by four circles of cloud-thunder patterns in triangles and sectioned with scenes of striking chimes music and feasting, hunting and naval and overland battles. There are designs of banana leaf patterns above the foot. The ring foot is decorated with cloud and thunder patterns in triangles. The vessel displays the exquisite casting skills and vivid patterns and pictures. It was collected in 1946.

Preserved in The Palace Museum

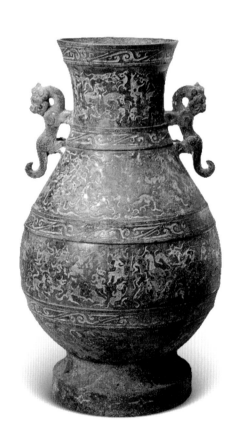

嵌红铜狩猎纹壶

战国前期

铜质

口径 14.7 厘米，宽 24.6 厘米，足径 16.7 厘米，

通高 40.7 厘米，重 4.82 千克

Pot with Red Copper-inlaid Designs of Hunting Scenes

Early Warring States Period
Bronze
Mouth Diameter 14.7 cm/ Width 24.6 cm/ Foot
Diameter 16.7 cm/ Height 40.7 cm/ Weight 4.82 kg

圆体，侈口，双伏兽纽，圈足，器身被四圈宽带纹饰分为四层，各层均饰狩猎图纹，宽带饰三角云雷纹，足饰菱形花纹。通体纹饰均以红铜镶嵌。1946 年入藏。

故宫博物院藏

The round body of this vessel has a flared mouth, two crouching beast-shaped handles and a ring-like foot. The body is divided into four sections by four circles of wide band-like patterns, and each section is decorated with designs of hunting scenes. There are designs of cloud-thunder patterns in triangles on the wide bands and diamond-like patterns on the foot. The decoration of the whole body is inlaid with red copper. It was collected in 1946.

Preserved in The Palace Museum

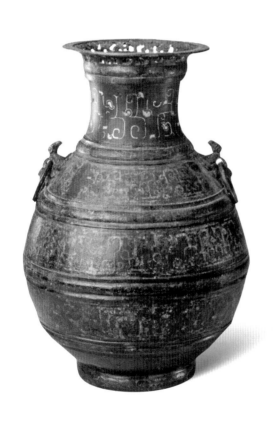

错金银鸟耳壶

战国前期

铜质

口径 17.4 厘米，腹径 26.1 厘米，足径 13.9 厘米，

通高 36.9 厘米，重 5.88 千克

Pot with Gold and Silver-inlaid Designs of Bird Handles

Early Warring States Period

Bronze

Mouth Diameter 17.4 cm/ Belly Diameter 26.1 cm/

Foot Diameter 13.9 cm/ Height 36.9 cm/ Weight 5.88 kg

圆体，硕腹，敛颈，圈足，伏鸟背带环双耳。
口卷沿平边，卷曲处镂空作兽纹，平缘上
饰绳纹；颈、肩、腹饰流云纹四道，纹饰
以金、银镶嵌，颈部纹饰除金银外，更以
绿松石镶嵌点缀，间隔花边及圈足上各饰
贝纹一周。清宫旧藏。

故宫博物院藏

The round body of this vessel has a big belly,
a contracted neck, a ring-like foot and two
ring-shaped handles hanging down from
crouching birds' back. The mouth is covered
with curled edge decorated with hollow-
out patterns of animals, while the flat edge
is decorated with cord patterns, The neck,
shoulder and belly are decorated with four
circles of floating-cloud patterns which
are inlaid with gold and silver. The neck is
also dotted with kallaite, and the alternative
lace edges and the ring-like foot are both
decorated with a circle of shellfish patterns.
The vessel used to be a collection of the
imperial palace of the Qing Dynasty.
Preserved in The Palace Museum

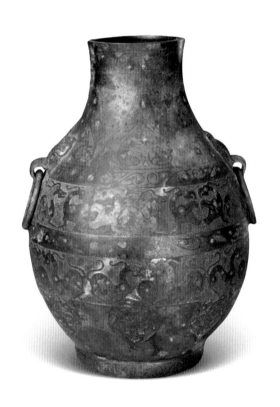

嵌红铜鸟兽纹壶

战国前期

铜质

口径 12.9 厘米，宽 27.7 厘米，足径 16 厘米，

通高 39.2 厘米，重 8.2 千克

Pot with Red Copper-inlaid Bird and Animal Pattern

Early Warring States Period

Bronze

Mouth Diameter 12.9 cm/ Width 27.7 cm/ Foot

Diameter 16 cm/ Height 39.2 cm/ Weight 8.2 kg

圆体，侈口，圈足，双兽首耳衔环。颈饰蕉叶纹；肩饰云纹；腹部正中以云纹一周将壶腹隔为二区，各饰鸟兽纹一周；腹下部饰蕉叶形纹一周，蕉叶内各饰双夔相盘纹；足饰云纹。颈、肩、腹、足云纹内以红铜镶嵌。清宫旧藏。

故宫博物院藏

The round body of the vessel has a flared mouth, a ring-like foot and two ring-shaped handles hanging down from beast heads. The neck is decorated with banana leaf pattern, and the shoulder is covered with a circle of cloud patterns which separate the belly into two sections. Each section is decorated with a circle of bird-like patterns. There is a circle of banana leaf pattern on the lower part of the belly, and inside of each banana leaf is decorated with a pattern of two Kui-dragons coiling up. The foot is covered with cloud patterns, and the cloud patterns on the neck, shoulder, belly and foot are inlaid with red copper. The vessel used to be a collection of the imperial palace of the Qing Dynasty.

Preserved in The Palace Museum

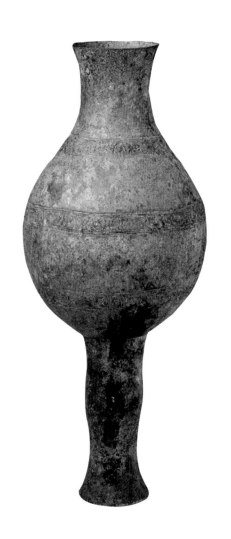

高足壶

战国后期

铜质

口径 4.8 厘米，宽 9.5 厘米，通高 22 厘米，
重 0.63 千克

Long Footed Pot

Late Warring States Period

Bronze

Mouth Diameter 4.8 cm/ Width 9.5 cm/

Height 22 cm/ Weight 0.63 kg

圆体，侈口，大腹，高足。腹部饰蟠虺纹

三道。1954 年收购。

故宫博物院藏

The round body of this vessel has a flared
mouth, a big belly and a long leg. The belly
is decorated with three circles of Pan Hui
patterns. It was acquired in 1954.
Preserved in The Palace Museum

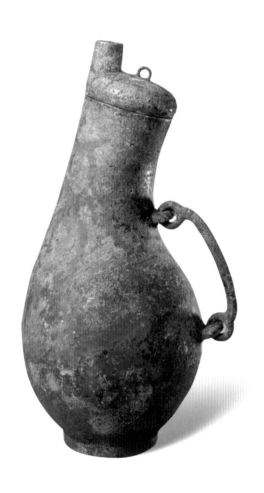

匏形壶

战国后期

铜质

口径 12.9 厘米，宽 20.3 厘米，通高 35.5 厘米，

重 2.12 千克

Bottle Gourd-shaped Pot

Late Warring States Period

Bronze

Mouth Diameter 12.9 cm/ Width 20.3 cm/ Height

35.5 cm/ Weight 2.12 kg

圆体，匏形，有盖，圈足。腹上有一活动
提柄，盖上有一桶状凸口。通体素无纹饰。
1959 年收购。

故宫博物院藏

The bottle gourd-shaped pot has a round body, a cover and a ring-like foot. The belly is equipped with a mobile handle. There is a bucket-shaped protruding mouth on the cover. The whole body has no any pattern. It was acquired in 1959.

Preserved in The Palace Museum

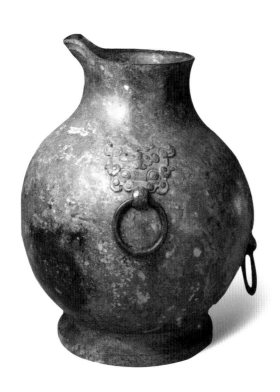

有流壶

战国后期

铜质

口径 17.9 厘米，宽 33.5 厘米，通高 38.3 厘米，

重 8.1 千克

Pot with Spout

Late Warring States Period

Bronze

Mouth Diameter 17.9 cm/ Width 33.5 cm/ Height

38.3 cm/ Weight 8.1 kg

圆体，大腹，圈足。肩有兽首衔环二，腹有兽首衔环一，口上有流。清宫旧物（原藏颐和园）。

故宫博物院藏

The pot has a round body, a big belly and a ring foot. On its shoulder and belly are respectively two and one ring-shaped handles hanging down from animal heads. There is spout on the mouth. The vessel used to be a collection of the imperial palace of the Qing Dynasty and was originally preserved in the Summer Palace.

Preserved in The Palace Museum

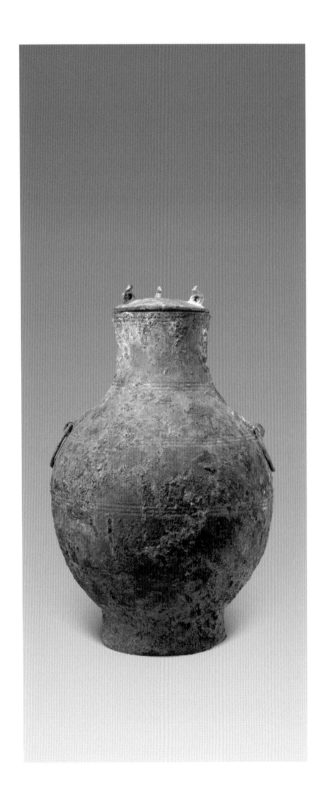

鸟纹壶

战国后期

铜质

口径 11 厘米，宽 24.7 厘米，通高 37.5 厘米，
重 3.48 千克

Pot with Bird Patterns

Late Warring States Period

Bronze

Mouth Diameter 11 cm/ Width 24.7 cm/ Height

37.5 cm/ Weight 3.48 kg

圆体，圈足，肩部二兽首衔环，有盖。盖上三纽，中饰涡纹；器颈、肩、腹上下饰浅雕鸟纹四周，间隔以弦纹。河南洛阳西宫秦墓出土，1956 年国家文物局调拨。

故宫博物院藏

The pot has a round body, a ring foot and a cover. On its shoulder are two ring-shaped handles hanging down from animal heads. There are three knobs on the cover with vortex patterns. The neck, shoulder and the upper and lower part of the belly are decorated with bird patterns in low relief, and alternate with string patterns. It was unearthed from the Tomb of West Palace of Qin Dynasty, Luoyang City, Henan Province, and allocated from State Administration of Cultural Heritage in 1956.

Preserved in The Palace Museum

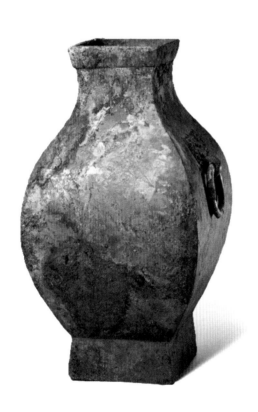

四升斜客方壶

战国后期

铜质

口径 17.2 厘米，腹径 20 厘米，通高 38.1 厘米，
重 4.9 千克

Four-liter Square-footed Pot

Late Warring States Period

Bronze

Mouth Diameter 17.2 cm/ Belly Diameter 20 cm/
Height 38.1 cm/ Weight 4.9 kg

中国古代青铜酒器。方体，方足，双兽首衔环，口下饰嵌铜三角纹，足外有刻铭 13 字。河南洛阳金村出土，1958 年收购。

故宫博物院藏

The square-footed pot has a square foot and two ring-shaped handles hanging down from the animal head. The mouth of the pot is decorated with copper-inlaid triangle patterns. There is an inscription of 13 characters on the outside the foot. It was unearthed at Jin Village in Luoyang City, Henan Province, and was acquired in 1958.

Preserved in The Palace Museum

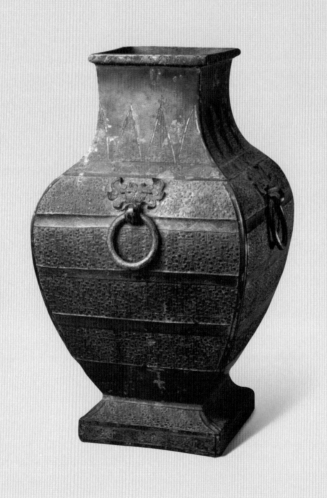

粟纹方壶

战国后期

铜质

口径 16.5 厘米，宽 31.5 厘米，足径 19.2 厘米，通高 49.4 厘米，重
12.72 千克

壶体作正方形，四兽首衔环。颈饰蕉叶纹，肩饰蟠螭纹一周，腹饰粟
状纹四周。清宫旧物（原藏颐和园）。

故宫博物院藏

Square-footed Pot with Millet Pattern

Late Warring States Period

Bronze

Mouth Diameter 16.5 cm/ Width 31.5 cm/ Foot Diameter 19.2 cm/ Height
49.4 cm/ Weight 12.72 kg

This square-footed pot has four ring-shaped handles hanging down from
the animal head. The neck is decorated with banana leaf patterns, and the
shoulder is covered with a circle of Pan Chi pattern. There are four circles
of millet-shaped patterns around the belly. It used to be a collection of the
imperial palace of the Qing Dynasty and was originally preserved in the
Summer Palace.

Preserved in The Palace Museum

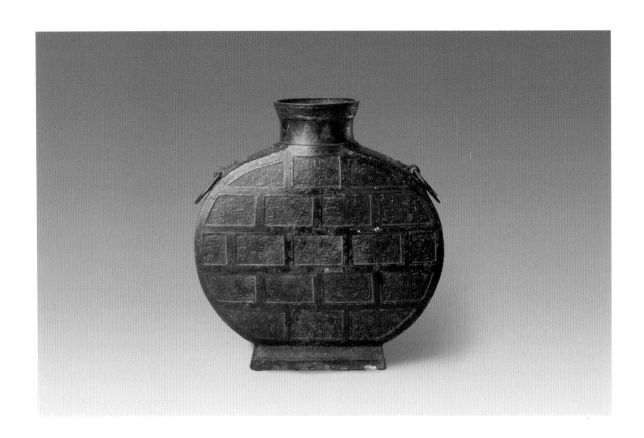

魏公扁壶

战国后期

铜质

宽 30.5 厘米，通高 31.7 厘米，重 3.96 千克

Oblate Pot with Characters "Wei Gong"

Late Warring States Period

Bronze

Width 30.5 cm/ Height 31.7 cm/ Weight 3.96 kg

扁体，长方足，肩部双兽首衔环。通身饰方格纹，方格内饰羽状纹。有刻划铭文8字，记此为魏公之扁壶，容积为三斗二升。清宫旧物（原藏颐和园）。

故宫博物院藏

This pot has an oblate body, a rectangular foot. On its shoulder are two ring-shaped handles hanging down from the animal head. The whole body is decorated with square patterns, and there are feather-shaped patterns inside the square patterns. This pot is inscribed with 8 characters, meaning that "This is the oblate pot of Wei Gong. The volume is 3 dou and 2 sheng" ("dou" and "sheng" are both Chinese units of measurement: 1 dou equals to 10 sheng, 1 sheng in volume measurement unit equals to 2 kg in weight measurement unit. In other words, this pot can hold 32 sheng in volume and 64 kg in weight). It used to be a collection of the imperial palace of the Qing Dynasty and was originally preserved in the Summer Palace.

Preserved in The Palace Museum

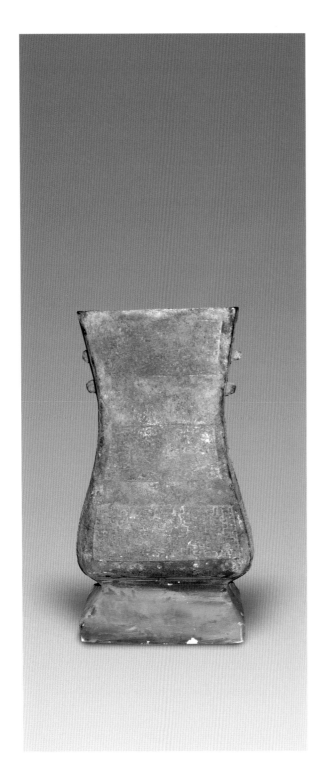

铜壶

战国

铜质

口径 13 厘米，底径 13.5 厘米，通高 25.5 厘米，
重 2.3 千克

Copper Pot

Warring States Period

Copper

Mouth Diameter 13 cm/ Bottom Diameter 13.5 cm/

Height 25.5 cm/ Weight 2.3 kg

方口，方腹，方底座，双乳丁耳。腹饰夔纹。
生活用器。底有修补。陕西省咸阳市废品
站征集。

　　　陕西医史博物馆藏

This pot has a square mouth and belly, a
square pedestal and two nipple-shaped ears.
The belly is decorated with Kui-dragon
patterns. This is a household ware. There are
complementary marks on the bottom. It was
collected at a scrapyard of Xianyang City in
Shaanxi Province.

Preserved in Shaanxi Museum of Medical History

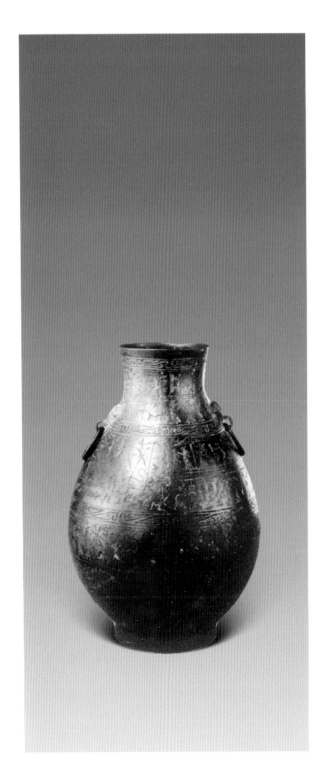

宴乐渔猎攻战纹铜壶

战国

铜质

腹径 24.6 厘米，通高 40.7 厘米

Pot with Patterns of Feasting, Fishing, Hunting and Fighting Scenes

Warring States Period

Bronze

Belly Diameter 24.6 cm/ Height 40.7 cm

侈口，敛颈，鼓腹，矮圈足。全器主体纹饰分三道：第一道表现射礼和后妃采桑；第二道为飨食礼、鼓钟击磬伐鼓等奏乐和弋射情景；第三道表现为水陆攻战场面。图像反映了战国时期贵族礼乐和戎事的情形。

故宫博物院藏

This pot has a flared mouth, a contracted neck, a swelling belly and a shot ring-like foot. The whole body is decorated with three streaks of patterns. The first streak of patterns displays the traditional shooting ceremony and picture of royal women picking mulberry leaves, the second streak of patterns shows the scenes of treating guests with food, feasting to music with striking musical bells, chimestone and drum, and hunting ceremony, and the third streak of designs includes the scenes of a land combat and a naval battle. These designs reflect the etiquette music and hunting ceremony of the royal family in the Warring States Period.

Preserved in The Palace Museum

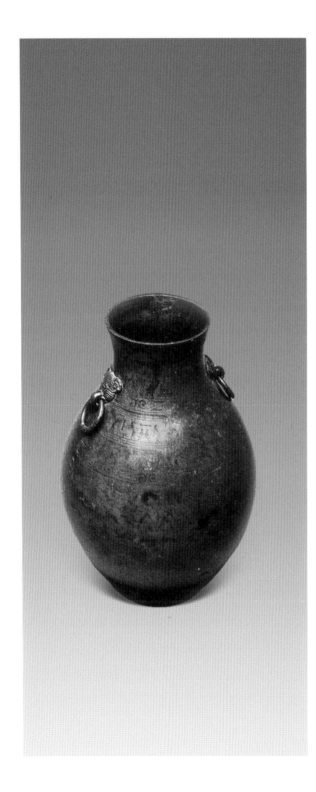

宴乐习射纹铜壶

战国

铜质

通高 32 厘米

Bronze Pot with Patterns of Feasting
and Hunting Scenes

Warring States Period

Bronze

Height 32 cm

长颈，圈足。肩部有两兽面衔环。壶身环布华丽的金属镶嵌错宴乐习射纹图案，主要内容表现的是一场礼射活动，周围还饰有宴乐、划船及狩猎等图案。

法国吉美国立亚洲艺术博物馆藏

This pot has a long neck and a ring-like foot. On its shoulder are two ring-shaped handles hanging down from the beast faces. The surface of the body is surrounded by gorgeous metal-inlaid scenes of feasting and hunting. These scenes mainly display a shooting activity. There are also some pictures about feasting, boating and hunting around the pot.

Preserved in Guimet Museum of Asian Art, France

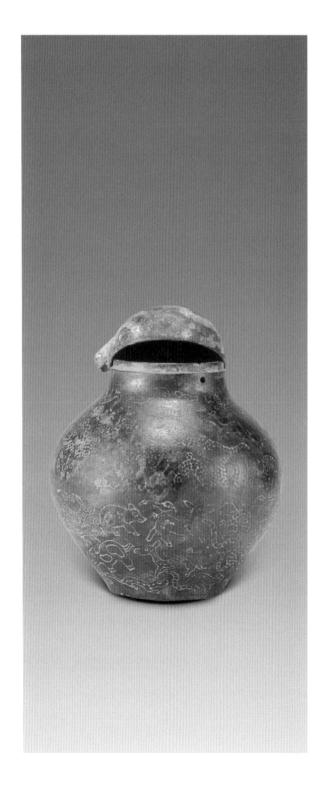

禽兽纹壶

战国

铜质

口径 4.2 厘米，腹径 9.5 厘米，底径 4.8 厘米，

高 11 厘米，重 0.4 千克

Pot with Fur and Feather Pattern

Warring States Period

Bronze

Mouth Diameter 4.2 cm/ Belly Diameter 9.5 cm/

Bottom Diameter 4.8 cm/ Height 11 cm/ Weight 0.4 kg

直口，短颈，鼓腹，平底，体为球形，口沿外有子母口和对称小孔，孔上器沿处有一小缺口，出土时上覆一半球形盖，其形如勺，盖素面。壶体外阴刻禽兽60余种。1982年陕西咸阳淳化县夕阳乡秋社村春秋墓出土。

淳化县文化馆藏

The pot has a straight mouth, a short neck and a swelling belly. On the edge of the mouth, there are a mother hole and symmetrical holes, and a small breach above the holes. When it was unearthed, it was covered with a hemispherical cover shaped like a spoon with no pattern. There are more than 60 animal patterns incised decorated on the body of the pot. It was unearthed from Chunqiu Tomb, Qiushe Village, Xiyang Township, Chunhua County, Xianyang City, Shaanxi Province, in 1982.
Preserved in Chunhua County Cultural Center

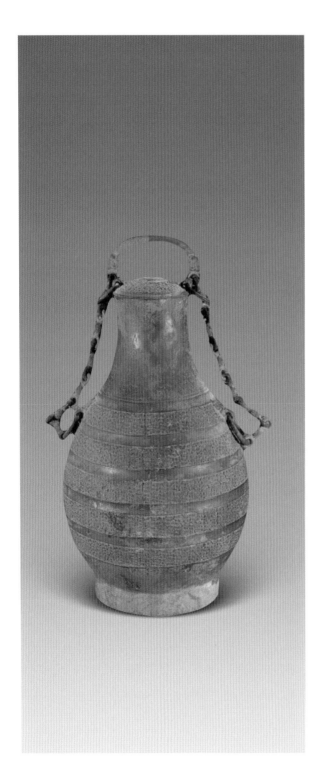

环梁浪花纹壶

战国

铜质

通高 37 厘米

Pot with a Looped Handle and Waves Pattern

Warring States Period

Bronze

Height 37 cm

器带盖，盖上有兽首提梁。壶直口，长颈，鼓腹，圈足。颈部饰一周蟠螭纹，腹部饰弦纹和浪花纹。两侧均有兽面衔环，每侧环上系有链索，向上与提梁连接。

河北博物院藏

This pot has a cover on which there is looped handle shaped into an animal head. The pot has a straight mouth, a long neck, a swelling belly and a ring foot. The neck is decorated with a circle of Pan Chi pattern, and the belly is decorated with string pattern and waves pattern. There is a animal mask pattern with rings in their mouth, and the ring on each side is chained to the chain cable which links the hooped handle.

Preserved in Hebei Museum

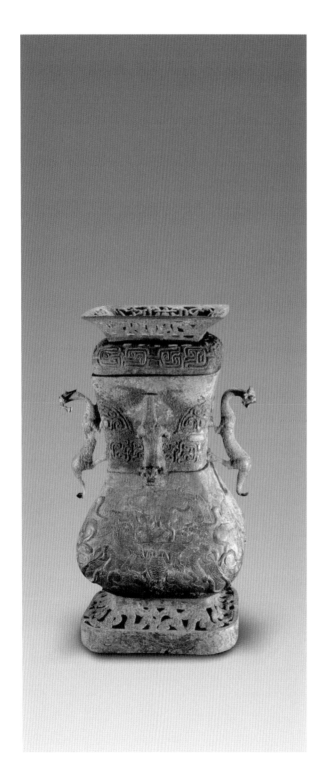

蟠龙纹方壶

战国

铜质

通高 51.5 厘米

Square Footed Pot with Pan-dragon Designs

Warring States Period

Bronze

Height 51.5 cm

直口，束颈，垂腹。委角方形盖，盖上部
为盘形捉手，盖下部的周边与颈部饰窃曲
纹。颈的四面均附虎形耳，虎的头部两只
向上，两只向下。腹部饰蟠龙纹和蟾蜍纹。
底座镂雕蟠龙纹和蟾蜍纹。

河北博物院藏

This pot has a straight mouth, a tightened
neck, a vertical belly and an eight-edged
square cover. There is a plate-shaped knob
on the cover. The lower part of the cover and
the neck are decorated with Qie Qu pattern.
All sides of the neck are decorated with tiger-
shaped handles, and the four tigers have two
upward heads and two downward heads. The
belly is decorated with Pan-dragon patterns
and toad patterns. The base is carved and
engraved with Pan-dragon patterns and toad
patterns.

Preserved in Hebei Museum

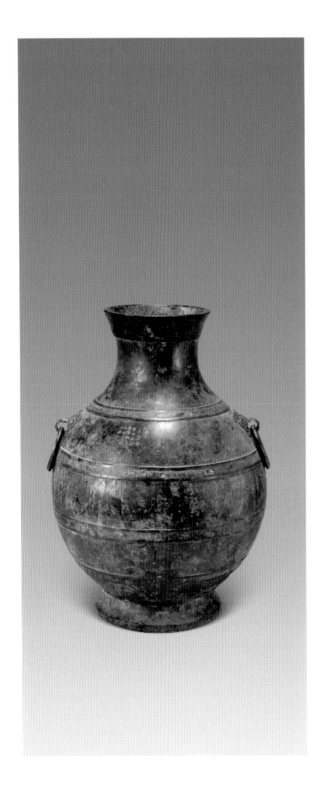

安邑下官钟

战国

铜质

口径 19 厘米，通高 56 厘米

Zhong with Characters "An Yi Xia Guan"

Warring States Period

Bronze

Mouth Diameter 19 cm/ Height 56 cm

器口沿刻有五字记容积"十三斗一升",
为秦人字体；颈部刻有"至此"二字，字
体为六国古文。该器记载了器名、造器年
月、官吏和器物容量。

咸阳博物馆藏

This vessel is inscribed with 5 characters on
the edges of the mouth，meaning 13 dou
equals 1 sheng (dou and sheng are units to
measure the volume). The neck is carved
with two characters "Zhi Ci". The vessel
recorded the name, manufacturing time,
officials and volume of this vessel.

Preserved in Xianyang Museum

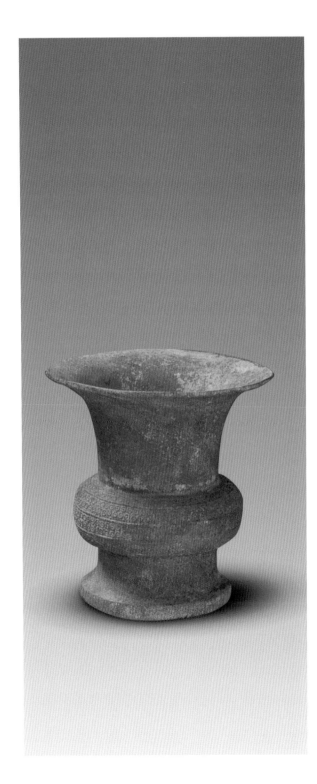

青铜尊

春秋

铜质

口径 15.4 厘米，底径 10.4 厘米，高 15 厘米

Bronze Zun

Spring and Autumn Period

Bronze

Mouth Diameter 15.4 cm/ Bottom Diameter 10.4 cm/

Height 15 cm

喇叭形，侈口，鼓腹，高圈足。腹部饰有四道弦纹，在弦纹中间有五条圈点纹带。这件青铜尊上的圈点纹曾见于南方商周时期的几何印纹硬陶上。溧水区白马镇上洋土墩墓出土。

南京市溧水区博物馆藏

This trumpet-shaped vessel has a flared mouth, a swelling belly and a long ring foot. The belly is decorated with four circles of string patterns, and there are five circles of circle-point patterns in the middle of the string patterns. The circle-point patterns on the bronze vessel once appeared on the hard pottery with patterns of geometric drawing in the south of Shang and Zhou Dynasties. It was unearthed at the mound tomb in Shangyang Village, Baima Town, Lishui District.

Preserved in Lishui Museum, Nanjing City

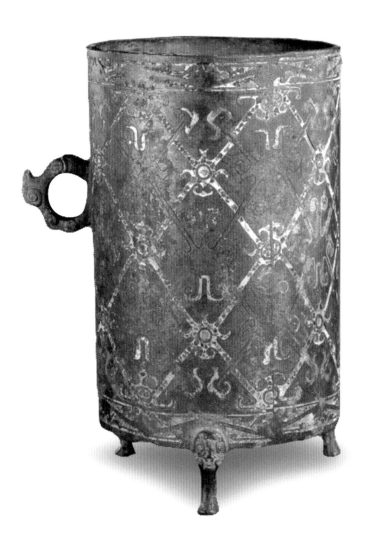

错金嵌松石樽

战国后期

铜质

宽 12.2 厘米，通高 15.3 厘米，重 0.66 千克

筒形，有环錾，三兽足，平底，把作鸟形，足上端作兽首。器通身以绿松石嵌成菱形、三角形纹饰，再以细线菱形错杂其间，细线菱形上下角错金为饰。1946 年入藏。

故宫博物院藏

Zun Inlaid with Gold and Turquoise

Late Warring States Period

Bronze

Width 12.2 cm/ Height 15.3 cm/ Weight 0.66 kg

This bucket-shaped vessel has a ring handle, three beast-shaped feet, a flat bottom and a bird-shaped knob. There are beast-heads on the feet. The whole body is inlaid with diamond-shaped and triangle-shaped turquoises, and alternated with diamond-shaped filaments. The upper and lower angles of the diamond-shaped filaments are alternately decorated with gold. It was collected in 1946.

Preserved in The Palace Museum

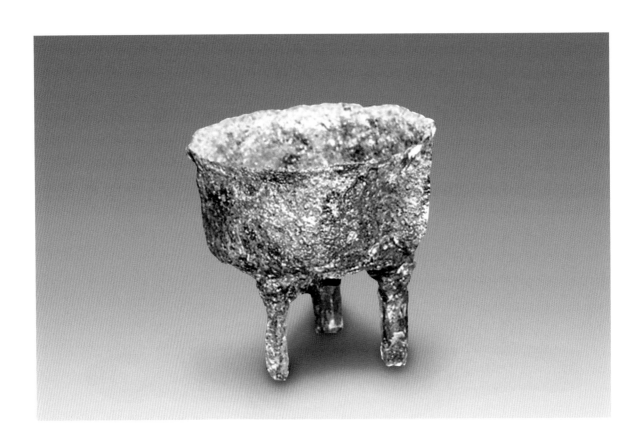

铁爵

战国

铁质

口径 5.5 厘米，通高 5.2 厘米，重 0.425 千克

Iron Jue

Warring States Period

Iron

Mouth Diameter 5.5 cm/ Height 5.2 cm/ Weight 0.425 kg

敞口，直腹，平底，三柱足全锈。酒器。有残。

河南省洛阳市征集。

陕西医史博物馆藏

The vessel has a flared mouth, an upright belly, a flat bottom and three rusty columnar feet. This vessel is used for keeping wine. There are damages to this vessel. It was collected in Luoyang of Henan Province.

Preserved in Shaanxi Museum of Medical History

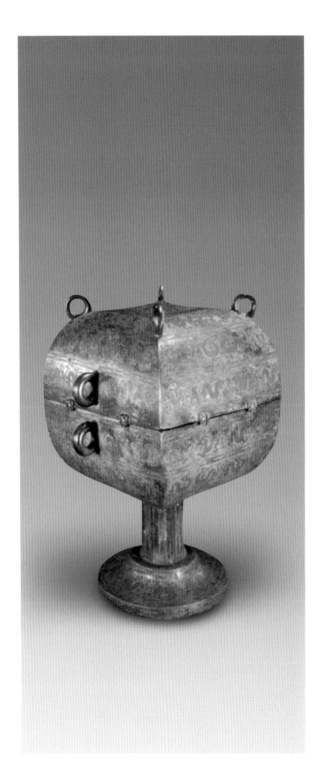

青铜方豆

春秋

铜质

长 7.3 厘米，宽 7 厘米，通高 30.5 厘米

Bronze Square Dou

Spring and Autumn Period

Bronze

Mouth Diameter 7.3 cm/ Width 7 cm/ Height 30.5 cm

此件主人季子系春秋末战国初宋国国君宋
景公之妹，于 30 岁左右早逝，这件铜豆
即系其陪葬品中的一件。河南省固始县侯
古堆大墓出土。

河南省文物考古研究所藏

This is a food container. The owner of this
vessel is sister of Song Jing Duke of the
State of Song in the Late Spring and Autumn
Period and early Warring States Period, and
she died young, about thirty years old. This
bronze vessel is one of her burial objects.
It was unearthed in the Hougudui Tomb in
Gushi County, Henan Province.
Preserved in Henan Provincial Institute of
Cultural Heritage and Archaeology

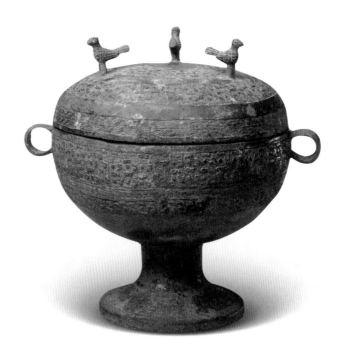

蟠虺纹三鸟盖豆

春秋后期

铜质

口径 18.6 厘米，通高 21.5 厘米，重 1.92 千克

Dou with Pan Hui Pattern and Three Birds

Late Spring and Autumn Period

Bronze

Mouth Diameter 18.6 cm/ Height 21.5 cm/ Weight 1.92 kg

大腹，高足，有盖。盖上饰三立鸟及绚纹
等三道纹饰；器身上饰绚纹等二道纹饰。
河南辉县出土，1958 年国家文物局调拨。

故宫博物院藏

This vessel is a food container, and it has
a big belly, a high foot and a cover. There
are three standing birds and three circles of
cord-like pattern on the cover. The body is
also decorated with two circles of cord-like
pattern. It was unearthed in Huixian County,
Henan Province and was allocated from State
Administration of Cultural Heritage in 1958.
Preserved in The Palace Museum

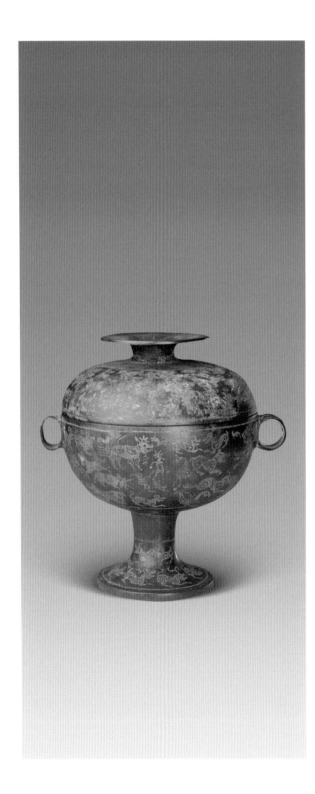

狩猎纹豆

春秋后期

铜质

口径 18.5 厘米，通高 21.4 厘米，重 2.22 千克

Dou with Hunting Pattern

Late Spring and Autumn Period

Bronze

Mouth Diameter 18.5 cm/ Height 21.4 cm/ Weight

2.22 kg

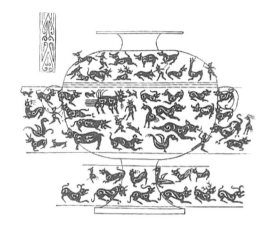

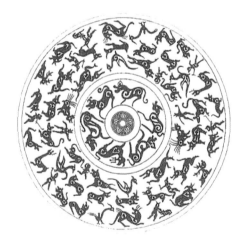

硕腹，作半球形，双环耳，高柄，圈足。腹饰嵌红铜狩猎纹，足饰鸟兽纹。清宫旧物（原藏颐和园）。

故宫博物院藏

This is a food container, and it has a big belly, a hemispherical body, two ring-shaped ears, a high rod-handle and a ring foot. The belly is decorated with red copper-inlaid designs of hunting scenes. The foot is decorated with fur and feature pattern. The vessel used to be a collection of the imperial palace of the Qing Dynasty and was originally preserved in the Summer Palace.

Preserved in The Palace Museum

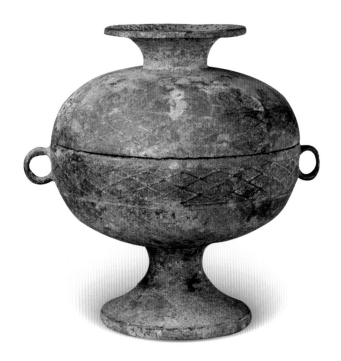

几何纹豆

春秋后期

铜质

口径 18.6 厘米，通高 21.5 厘米，重 1.92 千克

Dou with Designs of Geometric Drawing

Late Spring and Autumn Period

Bronze

Mouth Diameter 18.6 cm/ Height 21.5 cm/ Weight 1.92 kg

硕腹，高柄，圈足。腹饰对称的环耳。盖、
器纹饰相同，均以细密清晰的雷纹衬地，
上饰以嵌红铜的斜格纹。1958 年收购。

故宫博物院藏

This vessel is a food container, and it has a
big belly, a high rod-handle and a ring foot.
The belly is decorated with symmetrical ring-
like ears. The cover and body are decorated
with dense and clear thunder patterns against
copper-inlaid oblique grid patterns. It was
acquired in 1958.

Preserved in The Palace Museum

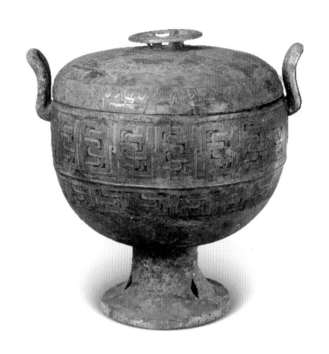

蟠虺纹豆

春秋后期

铜质

口径 35 厘米，通高 42.2 厘米，重 12.16 千克

Dou with Pan Hui Pattern

Late Spring and Autumn Period

Bronze

Mouth Diameter 35 cm/ Height 42.2 cm/ Weight 12.16 kg

大腹，双附耳，圈足，有盖，上有透空握。握饰雷纹，盖、腹饰蟠虺纹。河南辉县出土，1958 年国家文物局调拨。

故宫博物院藏

This vessel is a food container, and it has a big belly, two prick ears, a ring foot and a cover. There is a hollowed-out knob with thunder patterns on the cover. The cover and belly are decorated with Pan Hui patterns. It was unearthed in Huixian County, Henan Province, and was allocated from State Administration of Cultural Heritage in 1958. Preserved in The Palace Museum

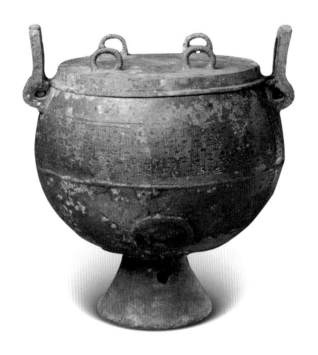

蟠螭纹豆

战国前期

铜质

宽 26 厘米，腹径 24.4 厘米，通高 27.8 厘米，重 3.4 千克

Dou with Pan Chi Pattern

Early Warring States Period

Bronze

Width 26 cm/ Belly Diameter 24.4 cm/ Height 27.8 cm/ Weight 3.4 kg

圆体，圈足，双附耳，有盖，盖平，上铸
有四环。盖顶及腹部各饰蟠螭纹一周，耳
上饰回纹，足有四穿孔，腹下部有三突起
痕迹。1954 年收购。

故宫博物院藏

This round vessel is a food container, and
it has a ring foot, two prick ears, and a flat
cover. There are four ring-like knobs on the
cover. The top of the cover and belly are
decorated with Pan Chi pattern. The ears are
decorated with rectangular spiral pattern. The
foot has four piercing holes, and there are
three protruding marks on the lower part of
belly. It was acquired in 1954.
Preserved in The Palace Museum

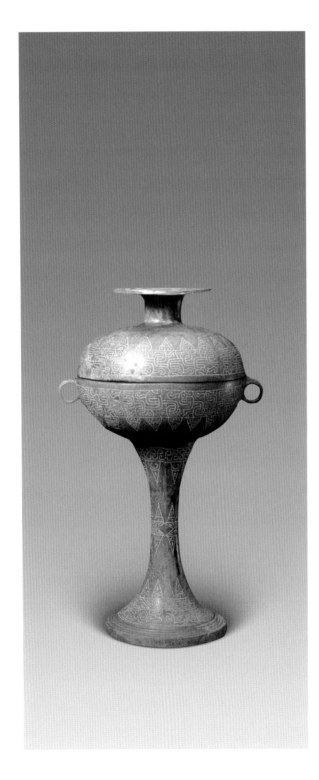

嵌松石蟠螭纹豆

战国前期

铜质

宽 24 厘米，通高 39 厘米，重 3.05 千克

Dou with Pan Chi Pattern Inlaid with Turquoise

Early Warring States Period

Bronze

Width 24 cm/ Height 39 cm/ Weight 3.05 kg

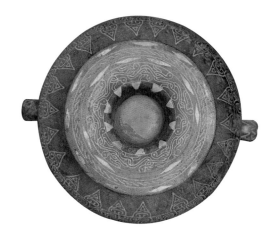

器束颈，两侧有环耳。盖顶有捉手，可以却置。盖、器饰嵌松石蟠螭纹，足上饰嵌松石垂叶纹，捉手饰菱纹，嵌饰颇为华美。1974 年顺义区东海洪大队出土。

故宫博物院藏

This vessel is a food container, and it has a contracted neck and a ring-like handle on two sides of the body. There is a knob on the cover, The cover can serve as another vessel when it is removed from the vessel it covers. The cover and the body of the vessel are decorated with Pan Chi pattern inlaid with turquoise. The foot is decorated with dropping-leaf pattern inlaid with turquoise. The knob is covered with diamond-like pattern. The inlaid decorations are gorgeous and beautiful. It was unearthed in Donghaihong brigade, Shunyi District in 1974.

Preserved in The Palace Museum

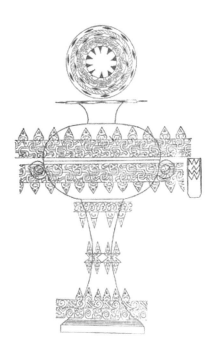

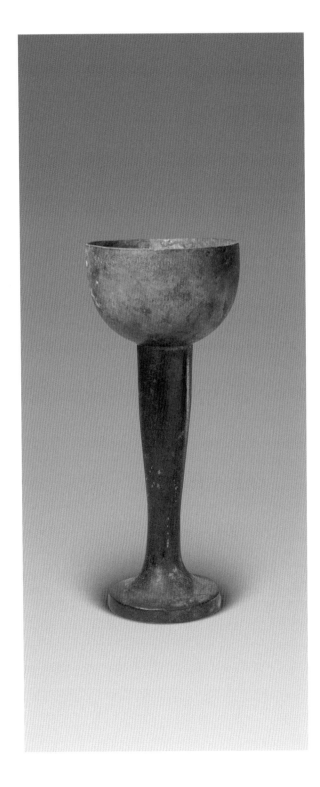

铸客豆

战国后期

铜质

口径 14.2 厘米，通高 30 厘米，重 2.34 千克

Dou with Characters "Zhu Ke"

Late Warring States Period

Bronze

Mouth Diameter 14.2 cm/ Height 30 cm/ Weight

2.34 kg

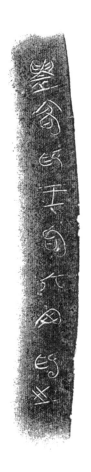

圆体，直口，高柱圈足，素无纹饰。器口沿有刻划铭文9字，记外方冶铸匠人"铸客"为王后六室做此豆。1933年安徽寿县朱家集出土，1959年北京市文化局调拨。

故宫博物院藏

This is a food container, and this round vessel has a straight mouth, a high columnar handle and a ring foot without any patterns. There is an inscription of 9 characters recording that the craftsman who named Zhu Ke made this vessel for the imperial harems which belongs to the queen. It was unearthed in Zhujiaji of Shouxian County, Anhui Province in 1933, and was allocated from Beijing Municipal Bureau of Culture in 1959.

Preserved in The Palace Museum

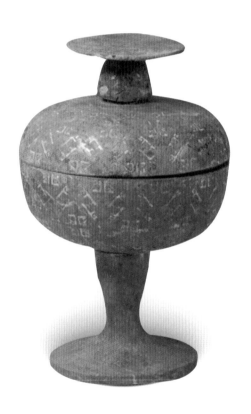

嵌金银铜豆

战国

铜质

口径 18.5 厘米，通高 25.7 厘米

Copper Dou with Patterns Inlaid with Gold and Silver

Warring States Period

Bronze

Mouth Diameter 18.5 cm/ Height 25.7 cm

盘为半球形，柄较高，喇叭形圈足，覆钵
形盖，扁平提手。盖面和盘外壁饰几何勾
连云纹，纹饰由黄铜丝与绿松石镶嵌而成。

山东博物馆藏

This plate is in the shape of hemisphere. The
vessel has a taller rod-handle, a trumpet-like
ring foot, a slip cover and a flat knob. There
are geometrical cloud patterns on the surface
of the cover and outer wall of the vessel. The
patterns are inlaid with brass fine wires and
turquoises.

Preserved in Shandong Museum

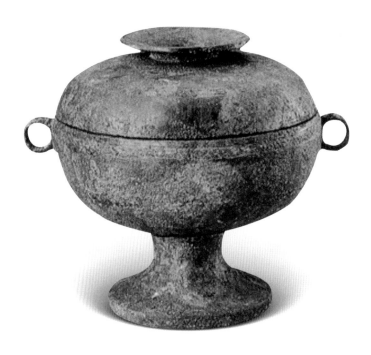

青铜带盖豆

战国

铜质

盘径 16 厘米，高 21 厘米

Bronze Dou with Cover

Warring States Period

Bronze

Disk Diameter 16 cm/ Height 21 cm

青铜豆盛行于两周，它既可以用来盛放干食如煮好的肉类，也可盛放调好的汤汁如羹类。在祭祀场合，豆是礼器之一，并是向神灵贡献牺牲的最后一道器具，即将肉从鼎中捞出在俎案上切好再置于豆中才可敬奉。在豆盘上加盖的组合流行于战国时期。

北京大学赛克勒考古与艺术博物馆藏

This Dou food container was popular in use in Western Zhou Dynasty and Eastern Zhou Dynasty. It was used for containing dry food such as cooked meat and mixed soup. Dou was one of the ceremonial articles in the sacrifice ceremony and the last vessel to offer sacrifices for god. Firstly, the ancients took out some meat from a cauldron, and then chopped it on a board. Finally, they could only put the meat into Dou to worship the god. The composition of plate and cover was a popular vessel in the Warring States Period. Preserved in Arthur M. Sackler Museum of Art and Archaeology at Peking University

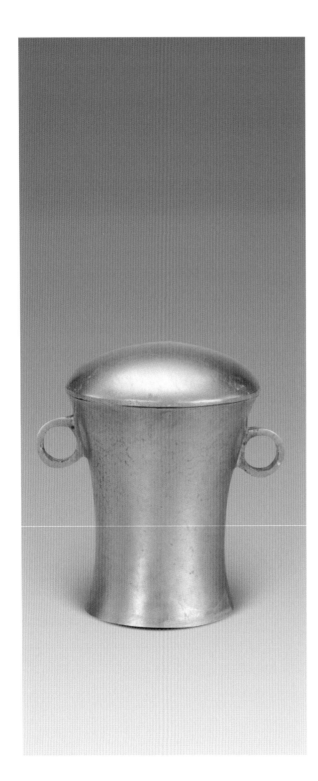

双环耳金杯

战国早期

金质

口径 8.1 厘米，通高 10.6 厘米，重 0.7899 千克

Gold Cup with Two Ring Ears

Early Warring States Period

Gold

Mouth Diameter 8.1 cm/ Height 10.6 cm/ Weight

0.7899 kg

饮食用器或酒器。敞口，平沿，杯腹上有两

个环形耳，平底。盖呈圆拱形，盖边上有三

个等距的御扣，可卡在杯内。通体光润，无

纹饰。1978 年湖北随州市曾侯乙墓出土。

湖北省博物馆藏

The cup was utilized as a food or wine
utensil. With open mouth and flat edge, there
are two ring-shaped ears on the belly of the
cup. The bottom is flat, the lid is circular,
and there are three equidistant handles on the
lid edge, which can be stuck in the cup. The
cup body is smooth with no pattern. It was
unearthed from Zeng Marquis Yi Tomb in
Suizhou City, Hubei Province in 1978.

Preserved in Hubei Provincial Museum

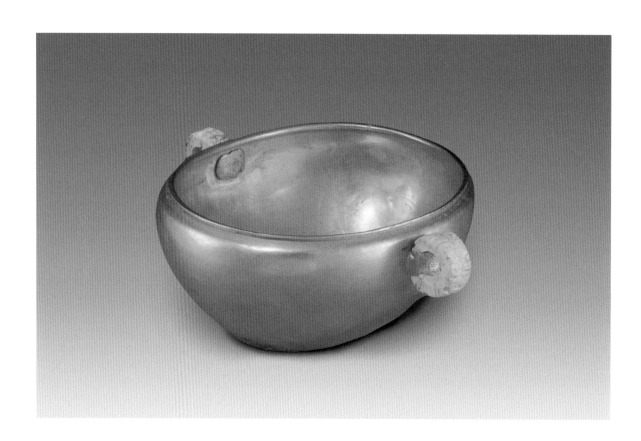

玉耳金舟

战国初期

器身黄金质，双耳玉质

口径 11.2 ~ 14.2 厘米，高 6 厘米，重 0.285 千克

Gold Zhou with Jade Ears

Early Warring States Period

Gold in Body and Jade in Ears

Mouth Diameter 11.2–14.2 cm/ Height 6 cm/ Weight 0.285 kg

舟身锻打而成，器表略显凹凸，敛口，卷沿，腹微鼓，呈椭圆形，平底。窄口部位对称铆接一对玉耳，呈环状。断面方正，琢刻精细卷云纹。同时期罕见的黄金器皿。

浙江省博物馆藏

The whole body is disposed of by forging and the surface of the vessel is uneven. It has a contracted mouth, a curled edge, a slightly swelling belly with the shape of oval, and a flat bottom. The narrow part of mouth is connected with a pair of ring-like jade ears. The fractured surface is upright and foursquare, and exquisitely carved with cloud patterns. It was a rare gold vessel in the same period.

Preserved in Zhejiang Provincial Museum

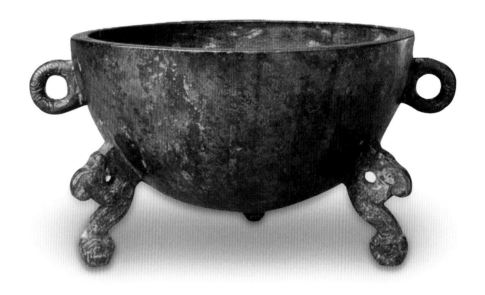

大府盏

战国后期

铜质

口径 23.3 厘米，通高 14.4 厘米，重 3.24 千克

Cup with Characters "Da Fu"

Late Warring States Period

Bronze

Mouth Diameter 23.3 cm/ Height 14.4 cm/ Weight 3.24 kg

器作半球形，三兽足，双圈耳，足作虺形，
虺首着地。器口上有铭文 5 字，记此器是
大府所用之盛盏。1933 年安徽寿县朱家
集出土，1959 年北京市文化局调拨。

故宫博物院藏

This domed vessel is in semispherical shape
and it has three animal-shaped feet, two ring-
like ears. The feet are made into the shape of
a snake, and the head of the snake touches
the ground. There is an inscription of 5
characters recording that this vessel was used
by "Da Fu". It was unearthed in Zhujiaji of
Shouxian County, Anhui Province in 1933,
and was allocated from Beijing in 1959.

Preserved in The Palace Museum

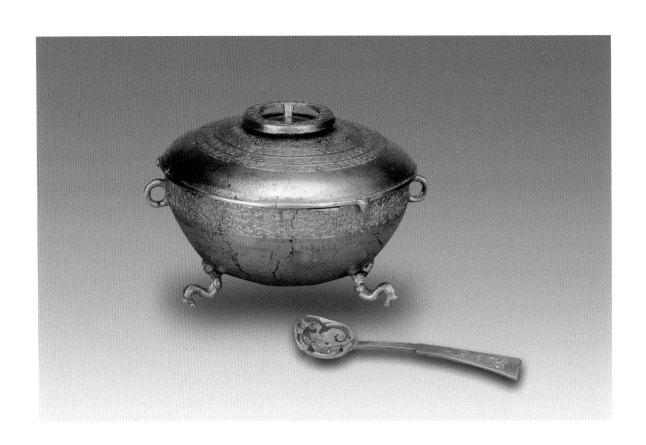

金盏、漏匕

战国早期

盏：口径 15.1 厘米，高 11 厘米，重 2.156 千克

匕：长 13 厘米，重 0.05645 千克

Gold Cup and Filtering Spoon

Early Warring States Period

Cup: Mouth Diameter 15.1 cm/ Height 11 cm/ Weight 2.156 kg

Spoon: Length 13 cm/ Weight 0.05645 kg

食器。盏全器饰蟠螭纹、绹纹、雷纹、涡
云纹等。匕面镂空成变异龙纹。1978 年
湖北随州市曾侯乙墓出土。

湖北省博物馆藏

They were utilized as food utensils. The
whole cup is decorated with Pan Chi pattern,
rope-like pattern, thunder pattern and cloud-
like pattern. The spoon is engraved into
hollow variegated dragon pattern. It was
unearthed from Zeng Marquis Yi Tomb in
Suizhou city, Hubei Province in 1978.
Preserved in Hubei Provincial Museum

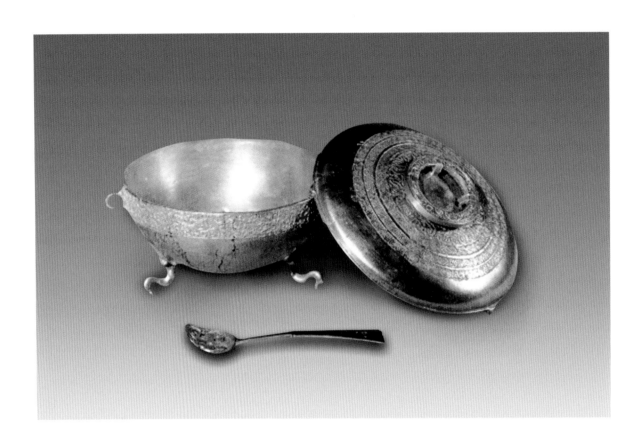

金盏与金匕

战国

金质

盏：口径 15.1 厘米，高 11 厘米，重 2.156 千克，纯度为 85% ~ 93%

匕：通长 13 厘米，重 0.05645 千克

Gold Cup and Gold Filtering Spoon

Warring States Period

Gold

Cup: Mouth Diameter 15.1 cm/ Height 11 cm/ Weight 2.156 kg/ Purity 85%–93%

Spoon: Length 13 cm/ Weight 0.05645 kg

此金盏为迄今所见先秦时期个体最大且最
重的金质容器。出土时，金匕放于盏内，
其功用为从汤羹中捞取块状食物。古代食
器。1978年湖北省随州市曾侯乙墓出土。

湖北省博物馆藏

This gold cup is so far the largest and heaviest
gold vessel in pre-Qin Period. The gold
filtering spoon was placed in the gold cup
when it was unearthed by the archeological
workers. The function of the spoon was then
for filtering lumpish food pieces from the
food soup. This is an ancient eating vessel.
It was unearthed in Zeng Marquis Yi Tomb
of Warring States of Suizhou City, Hubei
Province in 1978.

Preserved in Hubei Provincial Museum

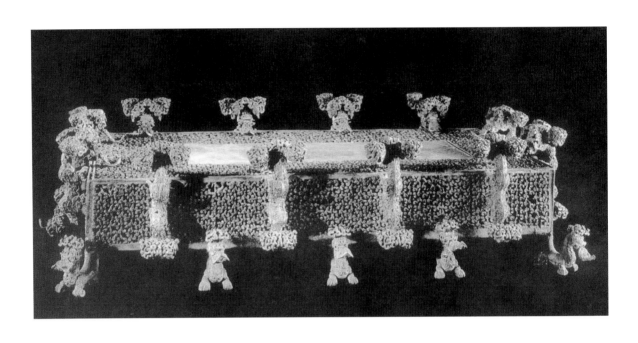

云纹禁

春秋

铜质

长 103 厘米，宽 46 厘米，通高 28.8 厘米

Jin with Cloud Pattern

Spring and Autumn Period

Bronze

Length 103 cm/ Width 46 cm/ Height 28.8 cm

器身呈长方形，中部有一个平面，平面周围及器身四壁均由镂空的、层层盘绕的云纹组成。12个昂首伸舌、挺胸凹腰的龙形怪兽支撑着整个器物。器身四周附有12个口吐长舌、曲身卷尾、攀缘登壁的龙形怪兽为装饰。禁是古代置放酒器的案子。1978年河南省淅川下寺2号楚墓出土。

河南博物院藏

This pedestal is in rectangular shape, with a plane surface in the center, the surrounding part of the plane and four walls of the pedestal are decorated with hollowed-out, coiled cloud-like pattern. The pedestal is supported by twelve dragon-like monsters which hold their head up, stick their tongue out, and hunch over. Surrounding the body is the decoration of twelve dragon-like monsters with twisted body and curved tails which stick out long tongues and climbs the surrounding walls. The pedestal "Jin" was used as the holder of wine vessels in ancient times. It was unearthed at Tomb No.2 of Chu State in Xiasi Village, Xichuan County, Henan Province in 1978.

Preserved in Henan Museum

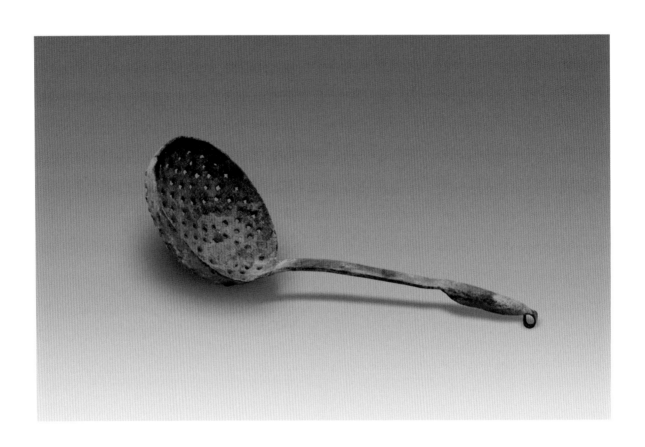

青铜漏勺

战国

青铜

漏勺：直径 10 厘米

手柄：长 26 厘米

Bronze Colander

Warring States Period

Bronze

Colander: Diameter 10 cm

Handle: Length 26 cm

漏勺布满均匀小圆孔，长执柄，尾端加粗，

环状耳。用于过滤中药汤液。

北京御生堂中医药博物馆藏

The colander has a long handle, a ring-shaped ear and bolded end, small round holes. It was used for filtering drugs of the traditional Chinese medicine.

Preserved in Chinese Medicine Museum of Beijing Yu Sheng Tang Drugstore

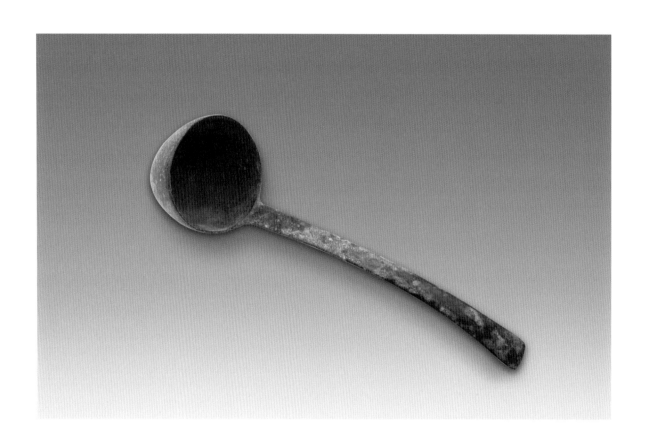

"吉羊"纹药酒勺

战国

青铜

径 6 厘米，深 8 厘米

Medicinal Wine Spoon with Characters "Ji Yang"

Warring States Period

Bronze

Diameter 6 cm/ Depth 8 cm

近椭圆形深勺头，长执柄，侧面有铭文"吉
羊"，寓意"吉祥"。盛药酒用。

北京御生堂中医药博物馆藏

The spoon has an oval head and a long
handle. The Chinese characters "吉羊" (Ji
Yang) are inscribed on the lateral side which
implies best wishes to people. It was used for
storing medicinal wine.

Preserved in Chinese Medicine Museum of
Beijing Yu Sheng Tang Drugstore

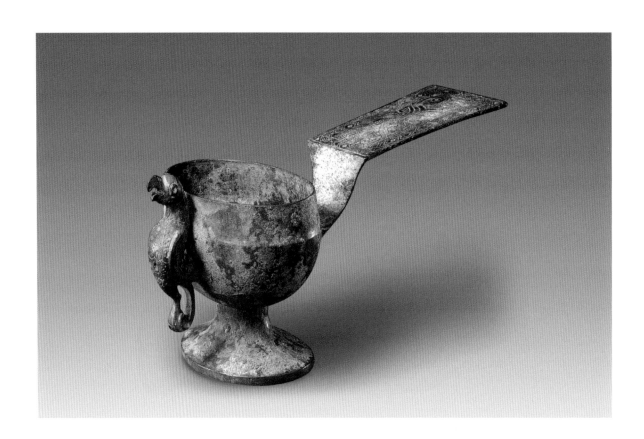

鸟饰勺

战国前期

铜质

口径 7.4 厘米，宽 16.5 厘米，足径 6 厘米，通高 8.4 厘米，重 0.2 千克

Spoon with Bird Ornament

Early Warring States Period

Bronze

Mouth Diameter 7.4 cm/ Width 16.5 cm/ Foot Diameter 6 cm/ Height 8.4 cm/ Weight 0.2 kg

勺体圆形，直口，圈足，腹壁外一端饰鸟
形饰件，另一端扁平柄，柄上刻有花纹。

故宫博物院藏

The body of the spoon is in round shape,
with a straight mouth and a ring-like foot.
One side of the belly wall is decorated with
a bird-shaped ornament, and the other side
is a flat handle with the decoration of flower
pattern.
Preserved in The Palace Museum

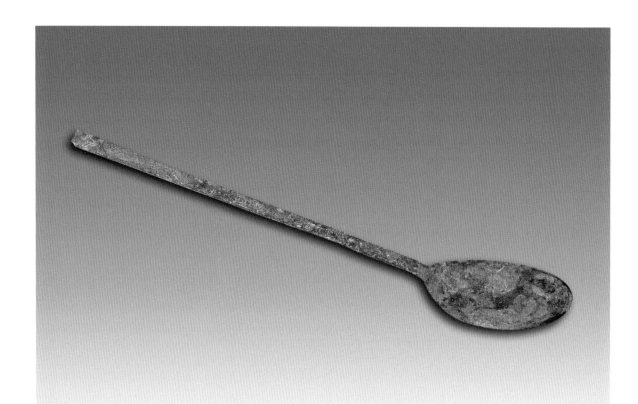

双鱼纹匕

战国后期

铜质

长 25.5 厘米，宽 3.8 厘米，重 0.5 千克

Spoon with Double-fish Pattern

Late Warring States Period

Bronze

Length 25.5 cm/ Width 3.8 cm/ Weight 0.5 kg

平勺直柄，勺内饰双鱼纹，柄面饰四鱼，纹饰均为单线刻成。1957 年国家文物局调拨。

故宫博物院藏

The spoon is in flat shape, with a straight handle and the inner area of the spoon is decorated with double-fish pattern. The surface of the handle is decorated with the pattern of four fishes engraved in single lines. It was allocated from State Administration of Cultural Heritage in 1957.

Preserved in The Palace Museum

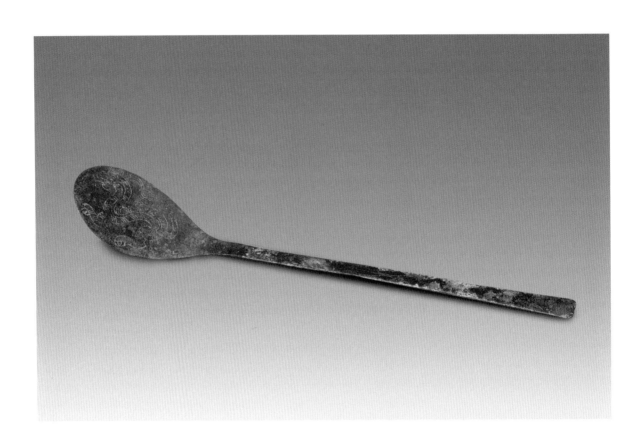

兽纹匕

战国后期

铜质

通长 21.6 厘米，宽 3.7 厘米，重 0.3 千克

Spoon with Animal Pattern

Late Warring States Period

Bronze

Length 21.6 cm/ Width 3.7 cm/ Weight 0.3 kg

匕前端圆，长柄。通体刻有花纹，匕端饰
一兽纹，兽张口立耳，有弯曲犄角，长身
弓背，两足，兽尾上翘。长柄上饰鱼纹，
刻划极细。1957 年国家文物局调拨。

故宫博物院藏

The front end of the spoon is in round
shape and with a long handle. The spoon is
decorated with flower pattern and the front
end is engraved with pattern of an animal,
opening its mouth, with prick ears and
curving horns. It has a long body, bended
back and two feet, with its tail curling up.
The long handle is decorated with very thinly
engraved fish pattern. It was allocated by
State Administration of Cultural Heritage in
1957.

Preserved in The Palace Museum

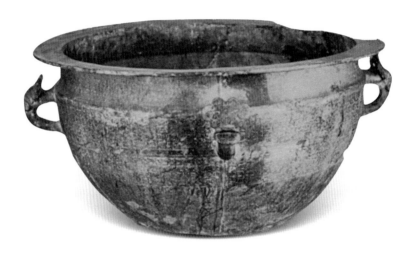

蟠螭纹四耳鉴

春秋

铜质

口径 62.5 厘米，通高 50 厘米

Four-eared Jian with Pan Chi Pattern

Spring and Autumn Period

Bronze

Mouth Diameter 62.5 cm/ Height 50 cm

敛口，宽平沿，束颈，弧壁深腹，平底。肩置四兽首环耳。颈饰勾连窃曲纹、勾尾蟠螭纹和空白相间三角纹，腹部饰蟠螭纹；四耳兽角镂空，当有衔环，环全失。盛水器或鉴容。

山西博物院藏

This is a water container, and it has a contracted mouth with wide and flat edge, convergent neck, a deep belly with cambered walls, and a flat bottom. The shoulder is attached with four animal heads with a ring in their mouth. The neck is decorated with connected Qie Qu pattern, Pan Chi pattern with coiled tails, and triangle pattern with blank margins. The belly is decorated with Pan Chi pattern. There are hollowed-out horns in the four animal head-shaped ears. There should have been rings on the four ears, which had all been lost. It was a water container or used to mirror one's face.

Preserved in Shanxi Museum

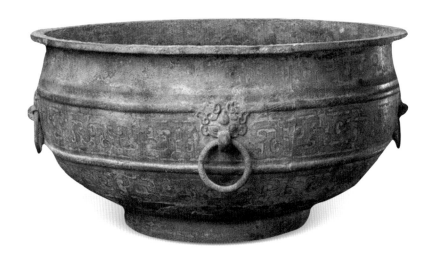

蟠虺纹鉴

春秋后期

铜质

口径 42.5 厘米，通高 34.3 厘米，重 5.6 千克

Jian with Pan Hui Pattern

Late Spring and Autumn Period

Bronze

Mouth Diameter 42.5 cm/ Height 34.3 cm/ Weight 5.6 kg

Relics of Chinese Medicine and Health (First Series)
Metal   Volume Two

口缘窄，束颈短肩；四兽耳衔环，两两相

对；腹部圜收，下有短圈足。腹饰蟠螭纹，

足饰贝纹。盛水器或鉴容。1957 年收购。

故宫博物院藏

This is a water container and it has a contracted
mouth edge, convergent neck and short
shoulders. There are four animal-shaped
ears with a ring held in the mouth on the
four directions of the belly. The round belly
extends inward, with short ring foot below,
and it is decorated with the pattern of Pan
Hui pattern. The ring foot is decorated with
shell pattern. It was a water container or used to
mirror one's face. It was acquired. in 1957.
Preserved in The Palace Museum

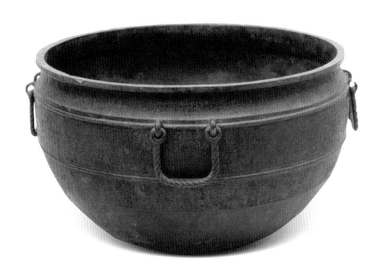

蟠虺纹大鉴

春秋后期

铜质

宽 61 厘米，通高 33 厘米，重 27 千克

Great Jian with Pan Hui Pattern

Late Spring and Autumn Period

Bronze

Width 61 cm/ Height 33 cm/ Weight 27 kg

窄口缘，束颈有肩，四个绚索耳两两相对，腹部圜收，底平。通饰蟠虺纹。清宫旧藏。

故宫博物院藏

This is a water container, and it has a contracted mouth edge, convergent neck and shoulders. The four ears with rope-like pattern confront with each other in four directions. The round belly, decorated with Pan Hui pattern, extends inward and has a flat bottom. It was originally preserved in the imperial palace of the Qing Dynasty.

Preserved in The Palace Museum

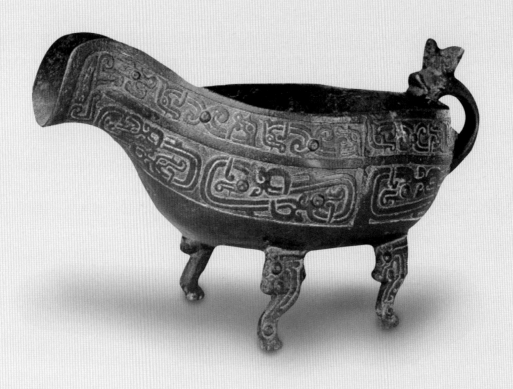

陈子匜

春秋前期

铜质

宽 29.8 厘米，通高 16.7 厘米，重 2.09 千克

口缘曲，流槽不甚长，腹较浅，龙形鋬，下具四条扁兽足。以蟠螭纹为主体纹饰。器内有铭文 5 行 30 字。盥洗注水器。1957 年收购。

故宫博物院藏

Yi with Characters "Chen Zi"

Early Spring and Autumn Period

Bronze

Width 29.8 cm/ Height 16.7 cm/ Weight 2.09 kg

This is a water container and it has a curved mouth edge, relatively shallow belly and a dragon-shaped handle. The water trough is not very long. It is mainly decorated with Pan Chi pattern. The inner side of the container is inscribed with 30 characters in 5 lines. It was acquired in 1957.

Preserved in The Palace Museum

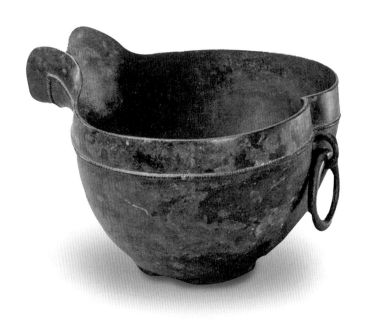

匏形匜

春秋后期

铜质

宽 40 厘米，通高 23.1 厘米，重 6.32 千克

Cucurbit-shaped Yi

Late Spring and Autumn Period

Bronze

Width 40 cm/ Height 23.1 cm/ Weight 6.32 kg

作半匏状。曲缘，短槽流；后部内收，錾
衔小环；下具三个扁长的矮足。口边饰有
一周绹纹。盥洗注水器。清宫旧物（原藏
颐和园）。

故宫博物院藏

This is a water container and it is in the shape of a half cucurbit. It has curved edge and a short water trough. The hind part of the container extends inward, with a small ring on the handle. There are three short and prolate ring feet below. The mouth edge is decorated with a circle of rope-like pattern. It was originally preserved in the imperial palace of the Qing Dynasty (It used to be a collection of the Summer Palace).

Preserved in The Palace Museum

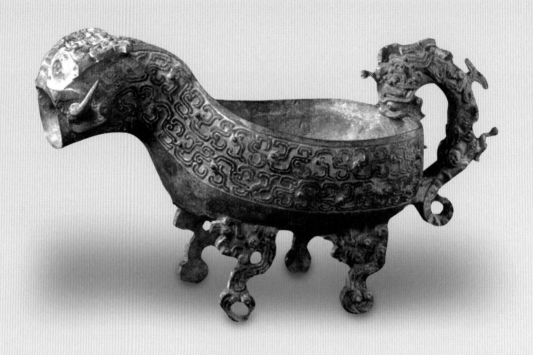

兽形匜

春秋后期

铜质

宽 42.7 厘米，通高 22.3 厘米，重 4.88 千克

兽头形曲管式流，浅腹，龙虎形鋬，间饰小兽，圜底下具四个扁兽足。器身饰蟠虺纹。盥洗注水器。1946 年入藏。

故宫博物院藏

Animal-shaped Yi

Late Spring and Autumn Period

Bronze

Width 42.7 cm/ Height 22.3 cm/ Weight 4.88 kg

This is a water container and it has a water trough with curved tube in the shape of animals. The belly is shallow. There is a dragon and tiger-shaped handle engraved with small animals. Under the round bottom are four flat animal shaped feet. The body is decorated with Pan Hui pattern. It was collected in 1946.

Preserved in The Palace Museum

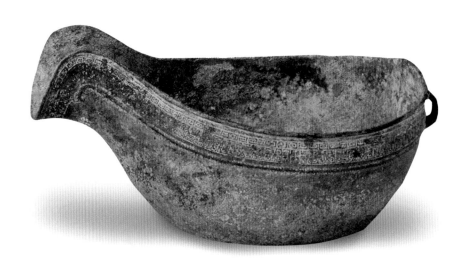

蔡子匜

春秋后期

铜质

宽 27.3 厘米，通高 11.9 厘米，重 1.1 千克

Yi with Characters "Cai Zi"

Late Spring and Autumn Period

Bronze

Width 27.3 cm/ Height 11.9 cm/ Weight 1.1 kg

曲缘，短槽流，浅腹，平底，錾为小圆纽形。口外饰雷纹和蟠虺纹。器内底 2 行 7 字铭文。盥洗注水器。国家文物局调拨。

故宫博物院藏

This is a water container and it has a curved edge, a short water trough, a shallow belly and a flat bottom. There is a small knob-like handle. The outer side of the mouth is decorated with thunder pattern and Pan Hui pattern. The inner area of the bottom of the container is inscribed with 7 characters in 2 lines. It was allocated from State Administration of Cultural Heritage.

Preserved in The Palace Museum

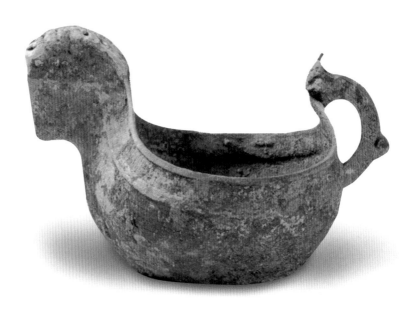

蟠虺纹铜匜

春秋后期

铜质

长 23 厘米，宽 20 厘米，高 14.5 厘米

Bronze Yi with Pan Hui Pattern

Late Spring and Autumn Period

Bronze

Length 23 cm/ Width 20 cm/ Height 14.5 cm

瓢形，宽扁腹，平底，流作管状，尾部有錾。腹部以绳索纹作间隔，饰二道宽带状蟠虺纹。流方口，上部镂空，饰蟠虺纹，作螭虎形。盥洗注水器。

南京市博物馆藏

The gourd shaped water container has a wide and flat belly, a flat bottom and a tube-like water trough. There is a handle in the tail end. Separated by the rope-like pattern, the belly is decorated with two streaks of wide belt-like Pan Hui pattern. The mouth of the water trough is in square shape. Its tiger-dragon shaped upper part of the water through is hollowed-out and decorated with Pan Hui pattern.

Preserved in Nanjing Municipal Museum

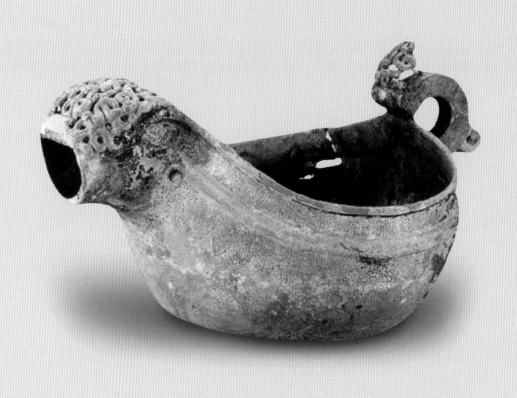

龙柄铜匜

春秋

铜质

通长 26.5 厘米，口宽 21.5 厘米，高 11.5 厘米

瓢形，圆鼓腹，平底，尾部有龙首状鋬。腹部以绳纹作间隔，饰宽带状蟠虺纹。流上部镂空，饰蟠虺纹，作螭虎形。盛水洗手用具。1972 年湖北襄阳山湾出土。

湖北省博物馆藏

Bronze Yi with Dragon-shaped Handle

Spring and Autumn Period

Bronze

Length 26.5 cm/ Mouth Width 21.5 cm/ Height 11.5 cm

The gourd-shaped water container has a round drum belly, a flat bottom. There is a dragon-tiger shaped handle in the tail end. Separated by the rope-like pattern, the belly is decorated with belt-like Pan Hui pattern. The dragon-tiger shaped upper part of the water through is hollowed-out and decorated with Pan Hui pattern. It was unearthed in Shanwan, Xiangyang City, Hubei Province, in 1972.

Preserved in Hubei Provincial Museum

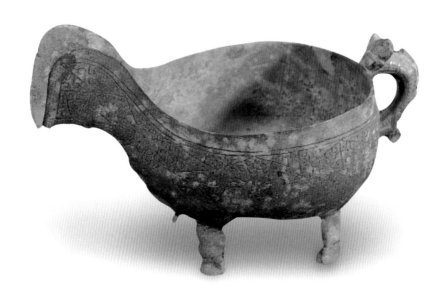

三角云纹"孟姬"匜

春秋

铜质

高 15 厘米

"Meng Ji" Yi with Triangle Cloud Pattern

Spring and Autumn Period

Bronze

Height 15 cm

敛口，深腹，敞口流，兽形柄，蹄形矮足。
器身阴刻三角纹，上饰卷云纹。

河北博物院藏

The water container has a contracted mouth,
a deep belly and open water trough. There
is an animal shaped handle and horseshoe
shaped short feet. The body is inscribed with
triangle patterns cut in intaglio, and the upper
part decorated with cirrus cloud-like pattern.
Preserved in Hebei Museum

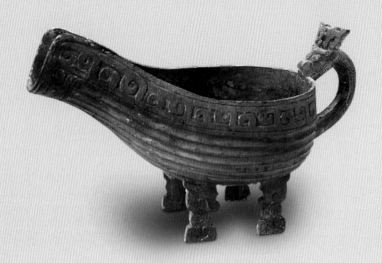

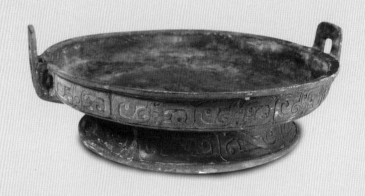

"樊夫人"盘、匜

春秋

铜质

盘：口径 35.5 厘米，高 13.3 厘米

匜：长 35 厘米，宽 16.1 厘米，高 20 厘米

Plate and Yi with Characters "Fan Fu Ren"

Spring and Autumn Period

Bronze

Plate: Mouth Diameter 35.5 cm/ Height 13.3 cm

Yi: Length 35 cm/ Width 16.1 cm/ Height 20 cm

盘浅腹，两耳，平底，圈足。腹外壁饰窃曲纹，圈足饰斜角云纹，两耳
饰重环纹。盘底铸铭文："樊夫人龙嬴自作行盘"。匜前部有宽流，后
有龙首状鋬，腹微鼓，底圜收，下有四条扁状鸟形足。口沿外饰带状窃
曲纹，流与腹下饰瓦纹，鋬外饰重环纹。底铸铭文："樊夫人龙嬴自作
行也（匜）"。盘和匜是一套盥洗器，通常是用匜注水于手，以盘承接
洗过手的水。1978 年河南省信阳干桥西出土。

河南博物院藏

The plate has a shallow belly and two handles, with a flat bottom and a ring-like foot. The outer wall of the belly is decorated with Qie Qu pattern, the ring-like foot is decorated with cloud-like pattern, and the two handles are decorated with multiple ring-like pattern. Both the bottom of the plate and the Yi is inscribed with 9 characters, meaning these two vessels were used for Mrs. Fan, named Long Ying, who was Queen of the State of Fan. There is a wide water trough at the front part of the "Yi" and a dragon-head shaped handle at the back part. The belly is slightly swelling, and the bottom extends inward. There are four bird shaped flat feet below the belly. The outside of the mouth edge is decorated with belt-like Qie Qu pattern, and the water trough and the outer surface of the belly bottom is decorated with tile pattern. The outer surface of the handle is decorated with multiple ring-like pattern. The bottom of the "Yi" is inscribed with 9 characters. The plate and the "Yi" form a set of containers used for washing hands. The "Yi" water container is used for adding water into the hands, and the plate is used as a water container to get the used waters flow down from Yi water container. Both containers were unearthed west of Ganqiao, Xinyang City, Henan Province, in 1978.

Preserved in Henan Museum

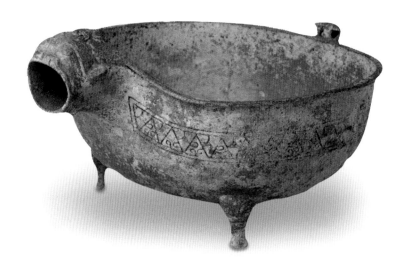

蛙纹匜

战国前期

铜质

宽 22.4 厘米，通高 11.5 厘米，重 0.68 千克

Yi with Frog Pattern

Early Warring States Period

Bronze

Width 22.4 cm/ Height 11.5 cm/ Weight 0.68 kg

造型独特，流作兽头形，兽头顶部饰有蛙
纹。屈舌兽首鋬，腹部饰双线勾边的三角
纹带。圈底下有兽足。国家文物局调拨。

故宫博物院藏

This is a water container, and it is uniquely
designed, with a water trough in the shape
of animal head which is decorated with frog
pattern in the top. The handle is in the shape
of an animal head with its tongue bended.
The belly is decorated with triangle pattern
belt with double-streak edges. There are
beast-shaped feet under the round belly. It
was allocated from State Administration of
Cultural Heritage.

Preserved in The Palace Museum

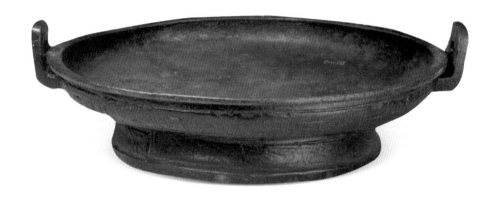

鲁伯厚父盘

春秋前期

铜质

宽 42.4 厘米，通高 12 厘米，重 5.64 千克

Plate with Characters "Lu Bo Hou Fu"

Early Spring and Autumn Period

Bronze

Width 42.4 cm/ Height 12 cm/ Weight 5.6 kg

圆形，折沿，附耳，圈足。腹饰窃曲纹，圈足饰斜角云纹。内底有铭文 10 字，记鲁伯厚父为其女儿仲姬俞做陪嫁用盘。1958 年收购。

故宫博物院藏

The plate is in round shape, with folded edge, two prick ears and a ring-like foot. The belly is decorated with Qie Qu pattern. The ring foot is decorated with cloud-like pattern. The inner bottom is inscribed with 10 characters. It was recorded that this container is a dowry which Lu Bo Hou Fu gave to her daughter Zhong Jiyu as a wedding gift. It was acquired in 1958.

Preserved in The Palace Museum

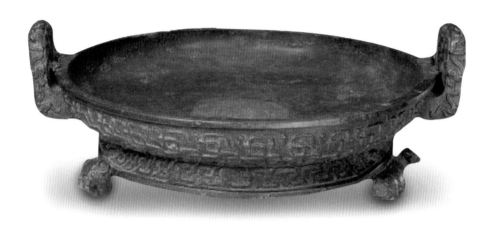

毛叔盘

春秋前期

铜质

口径 47.6 厘米，宽 52.5 厘米，通高 17.2 厘米，重 14.26 千克

Plate with Characters "Mao Shu"

Early Spring and Autumn Period

Bronze

Mouth Diameter 47.6 cm/ Width 52.5 cm/ Height 17.2 cm/ Weight 14.26 kg

敞口平缘，敛腹，外侈圈足下加饰三个牛
形附足。双耳起自腹部，上饰鸟纹和蟠虺
纹，腹、圈足均饰蟠虺纹。器内底有 4 行
23 字铭文。清宫旧物（原藏颐和园）。

故宫博物院藏

The plate has an open mouth, a flat edge, and
a convergent belly. The outward extending
ring foot is decorated with three cattle-
shaped attached feet. The two ears are on
the belly, and they are decorated with bird
pattern and Pan Hui pattern. Both the belly
and the ring foot are decorated with Pan Hui
pattern. The inner bottom is inscribed with
23 characters in 4 lines. It was originally
preserved in the imperial palace of the Qing
Dynasty (originally collected at the Summer
Palace).

Preserved in The Palace Museum

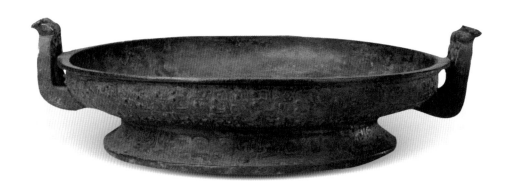

齐縈姬盘

春秋后期

铜质

宽 55.5 厘米，通高 15 厘米，重 11.39 千克

Plate with Characters "Qi Ying Ji"

Late Spring and Autumn Period

Bronze

Width 55.5 cm/ Height 15 cm/ Weight 11.39 kg

侈口，浅腹，圈足外撇。双附耳起于腹部，各饰有一对伏牺。以蟠螭纹为立体纹饰。器内底有 4 行 23 字铭文。清宫旧藏。

故宫博物院藏

The plate has a shallow belly and an outward extending mouth and ring-like foot. The two prick ears are attached to the belly, each of which is decorated with the design of a pair of crawling animals. The container is mainly decorated with Pan Chi pattern. The inner bottom is inscribed with 23 characters in 4 lines. It was originally preserved in the imperial palace of the Qing Dynasty.

Preserved in The Palace Museum

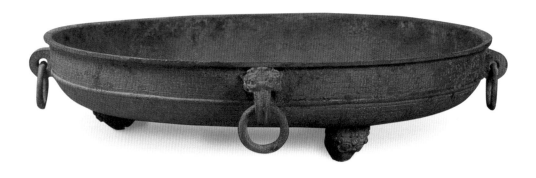

蟠虺纹铜盘

春秋后期

铜质

盘径 43.6 厘米，高 10.2 厘米

Bronze Plate with Pan Hui Pattern

Late Spring and Autumn Period

Bronze

Mouth Diameter 43.6 cm/ Height 10.2 cm

圆形，直口，方唇，浅腹，平底，底为三
兽面环形足。腹部以绳索纹作间隔，饰二
道宽带状蟠虺纹，腹上部铸衔环耳，耳饰
云雷纹、蕉叶纹及三角线纹组合。盘内正
中刻铭文1行，共10字。南京六合程桥出土。

南京市博物馆藏

The plate is in round shape. It has a straight
mouth, a square lip, a shallow belly and a flat
bottom. Under the bottom are three annular
feet in the shape of an animal face. Separated
by the rope pattern, the belly is decorated
with two streaks of wide belt-like Pan Hui
pattern. The upper belly is engraved with two
ears with rings combined with them. The ears
are decorated with the combination of cloud
and thunder pattern, banana leaf pattern and
triangle-streak pattern. The central inner
bottom is inscribed with 10 characters in 1
line. It was unearthed at Chengqiao County,
Liuhe District, Nanjing City.
Preserved in Nanjing Municipal Museum

嵌红铜蛙兽纹盘

战国前期

铜质

宽 41.7 厘米，通高 12.6 厘米，重 3.38 千克

Plate with Frog and Animal Pattern Inlaid with Red Copper

Early Warring States Period

Copper

Width 41.7 cm/ Height 12.6 cm/ Weight 3.38 kg

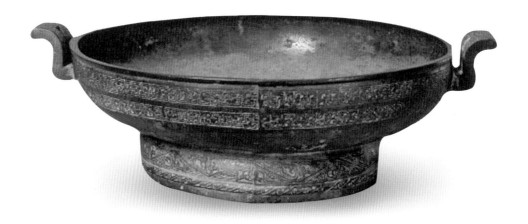

圆盘，圈足，双附耳。盘颈饰蟠螭纹二周；足饰三角夔纹一周，云纹一周；盘内底正中饰一"六星"纹，周围饰四蛙，外有八兽形纹；双耳饰动物纹。清宫旧物（原藏颐和园）。

故宫博物院藏

The plate is in a round shape. There is a ring foot and a pair of prick ears. The neck is decorated with two circles of Pan Chi pattern, and the ring foot is decorated with a circle of triangle Kui-dragon pattern and a circle of cloud-like pattern. The central bottom of the basin is decorated with "six-star" pattern, and the surrounding area is engraved with four frogs with the pattern of eight animals on the outer area, and the two ears are decorated with animal pattern. It was originally preserved in the imperial palace of the Qing Dynasty (originally a collection of the Summer Palace).

Preserved in The Palace Museum

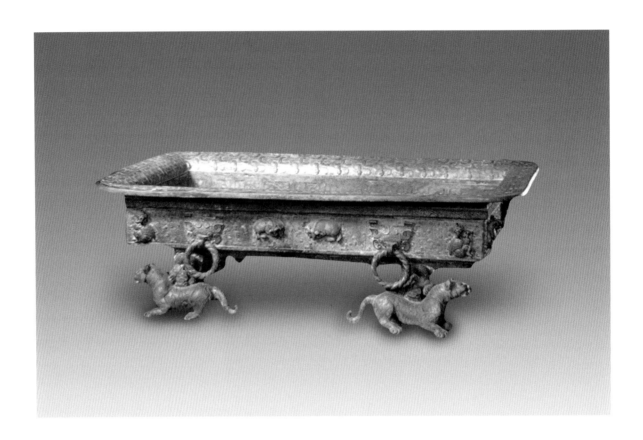

龟鱼纹方盘

战国前期

铜质

长 73.2 厘米，宽 45.2 厘米，通高 22.5 厘米，重 23.5 千克

Rectangular Plate with Turtle and Fish Patterns

Early Warring States Period

Bronze

Length 73.2 cm/ Width 45.2 cm/ Height 22.5 cm/ Weight 23.5 kg

长方体，口沿外翻，浅腹，平底，四兽首衔环，底部铸有四兽形足。宽口沿饰蟠螭纹，内底饰龟、鱼戏水图案，内壁饰曲带纹，外壁饰云纹及浮雕怪兽。清宫旧藏。

故宫博物院藏

The plate is in the cuboid shape, with its mouth edge extending outward. It has a shallow belly and a flat bottom. The outer surrounding walls are engraved with four animal heads with dangle rings in their mouth. There are four animal-shaped feet under the bottom of the plate. The wide mouth edge is decorated with Pan Chi pattern, the inner bottom is decorated with turtle and fish design, the inner wall is decorated with stripe pattern, the outer wall is decorated with cloud-like pattern and embossment of monsters. It was originally preserved in the imperial palace of the Qing Dynasty.

Preserved in The Palace Museum

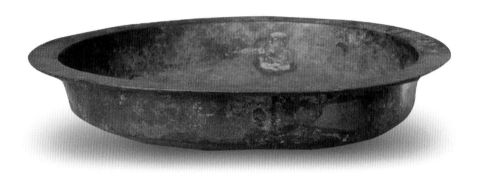

楚王酓忎盘

战国后期

铜质

口径 38.5 厘米，通高 7.9 厘米，重 3.08 千克

Plate of King of Chu with Characters Including " 酓忎 "

Late Warring States Period

Bronze

Month Diameter 38.5 cm/ Height 7.9 cm/ Weight 3.08 kg

浅盘无足，凸底平唇。素无纹饰。器口、
腹部各有铭文 1 行，口上 20 字，腹外 9 字。
1993 年安徽寿县朱家集出土，1959 年北
京市文化局调拨。

故宫博物院藏

The plate is in flat shape without feet. It has
a convex bottom and flat lip. The plate has
no patterns on it. The mouth is inscribed with
20 characters in 1 line and the outer belly
is inscribed with 9 characters in 1 line. It
was unearthed at Zhujiaji Village, Shouxian
County, Anhui Province in 1993, and was
allocated by Beijing Municipal Bureau of
Culture in 1959.

Preserved in The Palace Museum

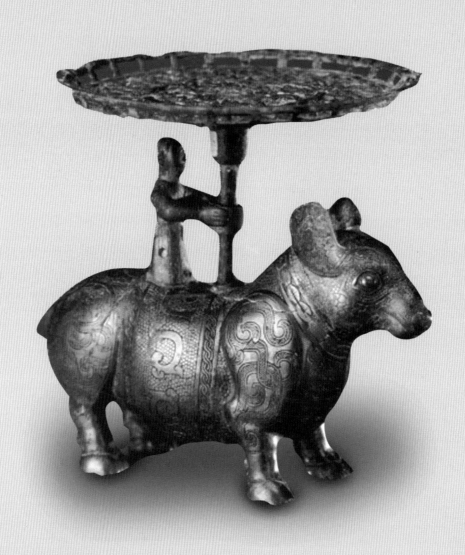

铜牺立人擎盘

战国

铜质

盘径 11 厘米，通高 14.6 厘米

铜牺造型为一昂首竖耳的怪兽，偶蹄，短尾。牺颈饰一周贝纹，身饰鳞纹，腹饰绚索纹与云纹，肩、臀饰卷石纹；牺背有一站立的女俑，束发垂肩，面目清晰，着右衽窄袖长袍，饰麻点纹，腰系带，双手前伸环握一圆柱；柱顶置一浅圆盘，盘敞口，平底，底部由形态各异的蟠虺构成镂空状，圆盘以圆柱为轴可灵活转动。盛食器。1965 年山西省长治市分水岭出土。

山西博物院藏

Bronze Plate Held up by Female Figure on an Animal

Warring States Period

Bronze

Diameter of the Plate 11 cm/ Height 14.6 cm

The bronze animal is a monster with prick ears, four legs and a short tail. The monster holds its head up high, and its neck is decorated with a circle of shell pattern. There are decorations of fish pattern on its body, rope pattern and cloud-like pattern on its belly, and coiled-rock pattern on its shoulder and hip. Standing on the back of the animal is a lady whose facial appearance is clear and has got bound hair reaching her shoulders. She wears a long gown of narrow sleeves, which is decorated with spot pattern. There is a belt on her waist, and she stretches her hand to hold the round pillar. On the top of the pillar is a shallow basin with an open mouth and a flat bottom. The bottom is decorated with the embossment of Pan Hui pattern in various shapes. The plate could flexibly rotate around the pillar. It was a food container which was unearthed at Fenshuiling Township in Changzhi City of Shanxi Province in 1965.

Preserved in Shanxi Museum

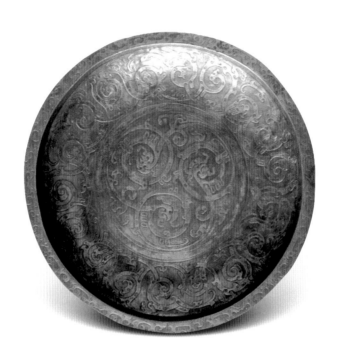

鎏金龙凤纹银盘

战国

银质

口径 37 厘米，高 5.5 厘米

Sliver Plate with Gilded Dragon and Phoenix Patterns

Warring States Period

Silver

Mouth Diameter 37 cm/ Height 5.5 cm

直口，平折沿，折腹，外底微内凹。口沿及内外腹壁各饰 6
组龙凤纹图案，内底饰 3 条盘龙，纹饰皆鎏金，线条流畅，
疏密适宜。器外壁与底刻有 "卅三年" 等铭文。盘上 "卅三年"
可能是秦昭王三十三年（前 274 年）所刻。汉灭秦后归汉，
又御赐齐王，故出自齐王陵的陪葬坑。盛器。1978 年淄博
市临淄区出土。

淄博市博物馆藏

The plate has a straight mouth, a flat folded edge and a folded
belly. Its outer bottom slightly concaves inward. The mouth
edge and the inner and outer wall of the belly are separately
decorated with six groups of dragon-phoenix pattern. The inner
bottom is decorated with three dragons which are decorated
with smooth gilding patters that are well arranged. The outer
wall and bottom of the plate are inscribed with the characters
meaning "the 33rd year", which might be inscribed in 33rd year
of King Qinzhao (274 B.C.). After the Qin State was replaced
by the Han Dynasty, this plate belonged to the Han kingdom
and was then granted to King of Qi State as a gift. That is the
reason why this plate was finally unearthed from the tomb of
King of Qi. It was a container and unearthed from Linzi District of
Zibo City in 1978.

Preserved in Zibo Museum

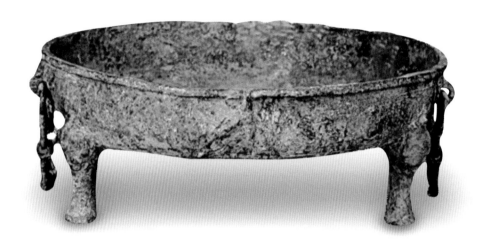

蟠螭纹三足盘

战国

铜质

口径 35.7 厘米，通高 13 厘米

Three-legged Plate with Pan Chi Pattern

Warring States Period

Copper

Mouth Diameter 35.7 cm/ Height 13 cm

敞口，窄平沿，浅腹，底近平，下承三蹄足。沿外两侧各置两铺首，套铸链环。腹饰蟠螭纹，足饰兽面纹。1954 年山西省长治市分水岭出土。

山西博物院藏

The plate has an open mouth, narrow and flat mouth edge and a shallow belly. Its bottom is almost flat and with three hoof-shaped feet below it. The two sides outside the mouth edge are separately decorated with two handles where there are chain rings hanging down from the handles. The belly is decorated with Pan Chi pattern, and the three feet are decorated with animal faces pattern. It was unearthed from Fenshuiling Township in Changzhi City of Shanxi Province in 1954.

Preserved in Shanxi Museum

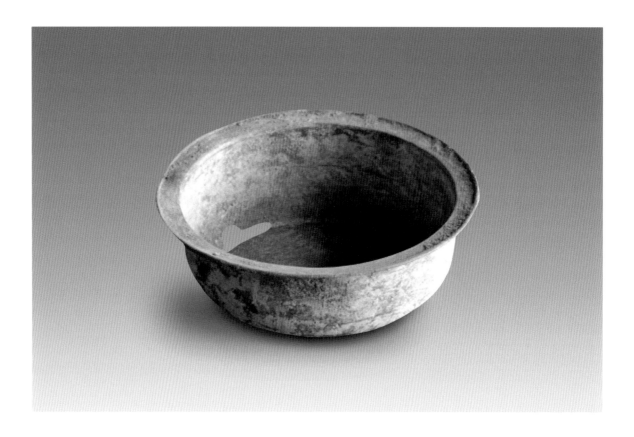

盆

战国

铜质

口径 21.5 厘米，高 7.5 厘米

Basin

Warring States Period

Copper

Mouth Diameter 21.5 cm/ Height 7.5 cm

宽沿，直腹，平底，底部残。成都市考古
队调拨。

成都中医药大学中医药传统文化博物馆藏

The basin has a wide mouth edge, a straight
belly and a flat bottom which is incomplete
for damage. It was allocated by the Chengdu
Archaeological Team.

Preserved in Museum of Traditional Chinese
Medicine Culture, Chengdu University of
Traditional Chinese Medicine

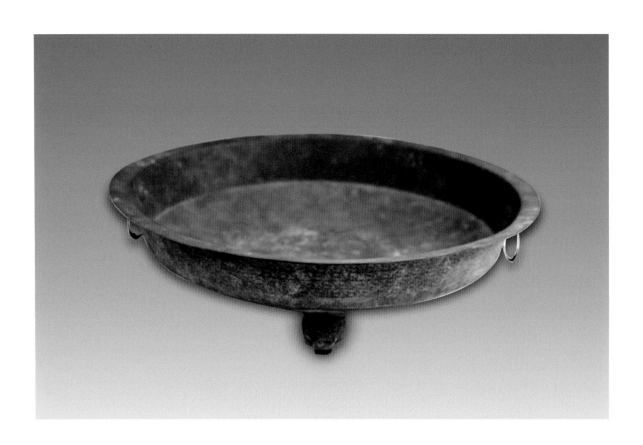

医工铜盆

战国

铜质

口径 40 厘米，高 12 厘米

Medical Copper Basin

Warring States Period

Copper

Mouth Diameter 40 cm/ Height 12 cm

敞口，外折沿，双环对耳，三足。专门用
来蒸煮药物或是用来消毒的器皿。

北京御生堂中医药博物馆藏

The copper basin has a flared mouth, a wide
folded rim, double ring-shaped ears and three
feet. It was utilized for decocting medicine
or disinfecting.
Preserved in Chinese Medicine Museum of
Beijing Yu Sheng Tang Drugstore

三足铜盆

战国

铜质

口径 39.5 厘米，底径 29.9 厘米，通高 15 厘米

Three-legged Copper Basin

Warring States Period

Copper

Mouth Diameter 39.5 cm/ Bottom Diameter 29.9 cm/ Height 15 cm

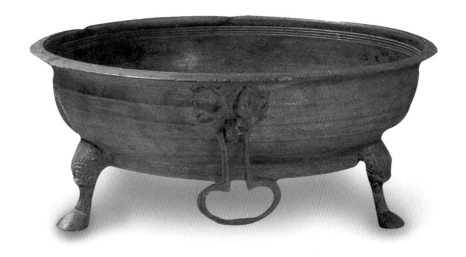

圆形，唇口外延，腹部微鼓，浅圜底，左右铸对称环把手。盆内壁饰阳线细弦纹五道，外腹部堆铸龙首衔环耳。器底附有三足，足铸浮雕兽首。

高淳区文物保管所藏

The basin is in round in shape, with its mouth edge extending outward and the belly slightly swelling. The bottom is shallow and round. There are two ring-like handles on each side of the belly. The inner wall of the basin is decorated with five streaks of thin string pattern. The outer belly is inscribed with a pair of ears which are in the shape of dragon head holding rings in their mouth. There are three legs under the bottom, which are inscribed with embossment of animal heads.

Preserved in The Institute for Cultural Relics Preservation at Gaochun District

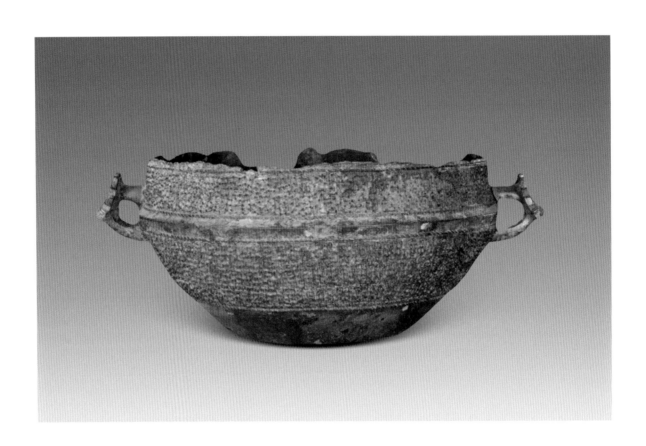

娄君盂

春秋后期

铜质

宽 33.2 厘米，通高 12.8 厘米，重 2.28 千克

Caverna with Characters "Lou Jun"

Late Spring and Autumn Period

Bronze

Width 33.2 cm/ Height 12.8 cm/ Weight 2.28 kg

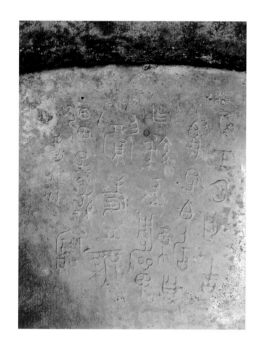

敛颈，折肩，腹圜收，平底。肩上有二兽耳。颈、腹均饰上下两周绚纹，各填以刺状蟠虺纹。器内底有铭文 6 行 26 字。传此器得于河南项城，1959 年浙江省博物馆拨赠。

故宫博物院藏

This container has a convergent neck, a folded shoulder and a flat bottom. Its belly is slightly contracted inward. There are two animal-shaped ears on each side of its shoulder. The neck and belly are all decorated with two streaks of rope pattern from the upper part to the bottom, and combines with Pan Hui pattern. The inner bottom of the container is inscribed with 26 characters in 6 lines. It is said that this container was unearthed from Xiangcheng City of Henan Province, and it was donated by Zhejiang Provincial Museum in 1959.

Preserved in The Palace Museum

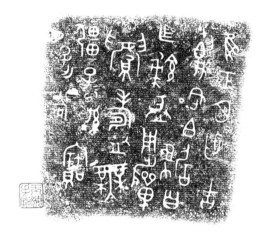

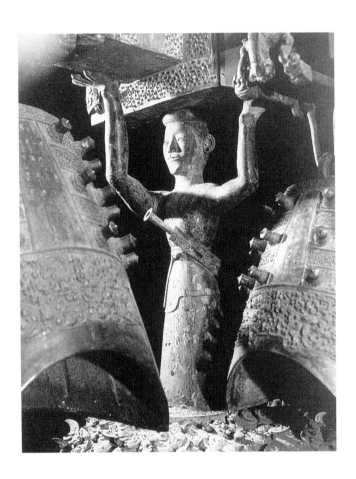

擎钟架青铜力士

战国

铜质

通高约 117 厘米

Bronze Herakles Holding up the Chime Bells and Rack

Warring States Period

Bronze

Height 117 cm

这一青铜力士为重达 2500 多千克大型编钟及钟架的承重立柱。其通身漆以彩绘，面部表情庄严，腰际佩剑，双臂上举，承托着编钟的横梁。整个造型给人以气势庄严肃穆之感。1978 年湖北省随州市雷鼓墩曾侯乙墓出土。

湖北省博物馆藏

This bronze Herakles is a supporting pillar which bears the weight of heavier tham 2500 kg of large chime bells and its rack. The whole body of the Herakles is painted with colored drawing, and its facial expression is dignified. With a sword wore at his waist, the Herakles raises up his two arms and supports the beam of the chime bells. The whole designing and shape presents us with a sense of solemnity. It was unearthed from Zeng Marquis Yi Tomb of Leigudun in Suizhou City, Hubei Province in 1978.
Preserved in Hubei Provincial Museum

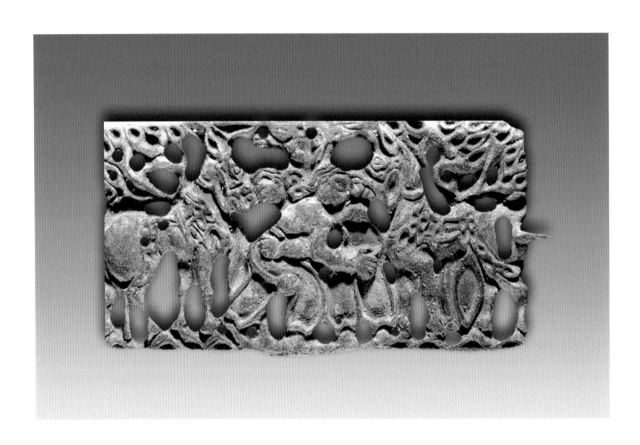

角抵图铜饰牌

战国

铜质

长 13.8 厘米，宽 7.1 厘米

Copper Board with Decorations of Ancient Wrestling Scenes

Warring States Period

Bronze

Length 13.8 cm/ Width 7.1 cm

铜饰牌为长方形，上面的角抵图为透雕而成。画面描绘的是在茂密的林木中进行的一场角抵比赛：比赛双方均赤裸上身，下穿短裤，左边的人用右手搂住对方的腰部，左手抓紧对方的后胯；右边的人用两手分别抱住对手的腰部和右腿。双方相持不下，都想极力摔倒对方，夺取胜利。画面背景的林木中，有二人骑乘的骏马，使饰牌的构图更具情趣。1955 年陕西省西安市长安区客省庄出土。

陕西历史博物馆藏

The copper board is in rectangular shape, which is engraved with the embossment of ancient wrestling scenes: we can see from the picture that the wrestling competition is held in the forest, the two wrestlers are all naked to the waist and wear shorts. The one on the left holds the waist of the other one in his arms with the right hand, and firmly grasps his opponent's back hip with the left hand. The one on the right holds his opponent's waist and right leg in his arms. Both of them refuse to yield, and they both want to defeat each other and win the competition. On the background of the picture are their beautiful horses, which make the decoration and arrangement of the board more vivid and interesting. It was unearthed in Kesheng Village of Chang'an District of Xi'an in Shaanxi Province in 1955.

Preserved in Shaanxi History Museum

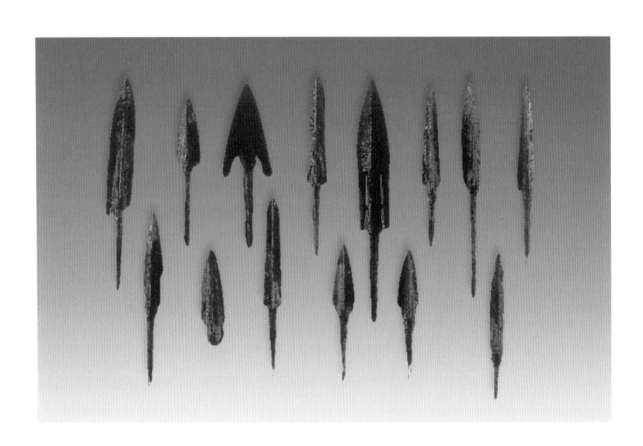

铜箭镞

战国

铜质

连杆长 67~71 厘米，直径 0.4~0.7 厘米

Copper Arrowheads

Warring States Period

Bronze

Length 67–71 cm/ Diameter 0.4–0.7 cm

铜镞分双翼形、三棱形、方锥形和圆锥形
四种形态，为战国时期射箭活动中常见的
箭镞形式。1978 年湖北省随州市擂鼓墩
曾侯乙墓出土。

湖北省博物馆藏

These copper arrowheads are in twin blades,
prismatic shape, quadrate-shaped form and
cone-shaped form, which are the common
styles of arrowheads in the Warring States
Period. It was unearthed from Zeng Marquis
Yi Tomb of Leigudun in Suizhou City, Hubei
Province in 1978.

Preserved in Hubei Provincial Museum

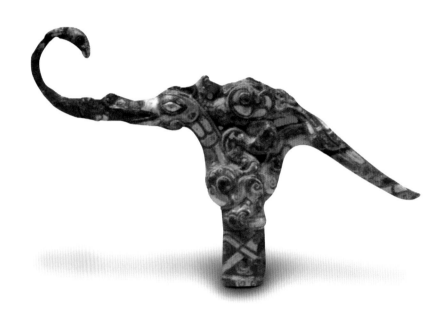

嵌金镶银铜杖首

战国

金镶银质

高 10.5 厘米

Copper Crutch Head Inlaid with Silver and Gold

Warring States Period

Silver inlaid with gold

Height 10.5 cm

鸟形。大鸟背负一小鸟，口衔一长颈鸟，鸟回首反顾。器下部为圆筒形銎，内有朽木。通体错金银。

曲阜市文物局藏

This crutch is in the shape of birds. The big bird carries a small one on its back, and by its mouth another bird of long neck that turns its head back to look. The lower part of the crutch head is a round shaped hole for installing a handle. There is rotten wood inside the hole. The whole crutch head is smeared with silver and gold.

Preserved in Qufu Bureau of Cultural Relics

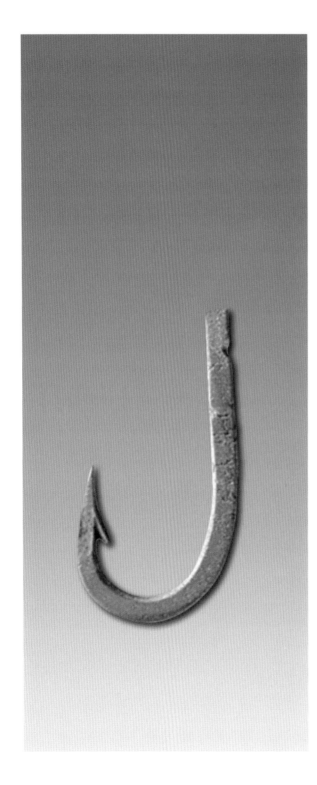

青铜钓钩

春秋战国

铜质

长 2.7 厘米

Bronze Hook

Spring-autumn and Warning States Period

Copper

Length 2.7 cm

钩身断面扁方，钩尖有清晰的锉痕。

浙江省文物考古研究所藏

The hook has a flat and square shaped fault plane in its body part. There is clear filing trace in the hook tip.

Preserved in Institute of Cultural Relics and Archaeology of Zhejiang Province

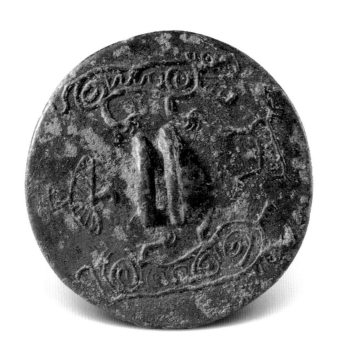

鸟兽纹镜

春秋早期

铜质

径 6.7 厘米

Mirror with Fur and Feather Patterns

Early Spring and Autumn Period

Copper

Diameter 6.7 cm

弓形纽。纽上方为一张口翘尾、头有双角竖立的小鹿，下方饰一展翅飞翔的鸟纹，左右各饰一虎，张口露齿，足向上屈，利爪张开。纹饰用阳线勾勒。1957 年河南三门峡上村岭出土。

中国国家博物馆藏

The mirror has an arch-shaped knob. On the top of the knob, there is a deerlet with upright horns on its head and that curls up its tail. Below the knob is the pattern of a flying bird. The right and left side are separately decorated with two tigers which open their mouth and sharp claws. Their feet bend upward. All the patterns are sketched out with protruding streaks. It was unearthed from Shangcunling, Sanmenxia City, Henan Province.

Preserved in National Museum of China

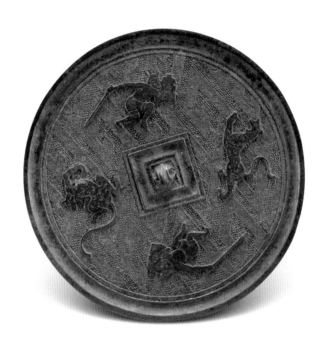

狩猎纹镜

战国

铜质

径 10.4 厘米

Mirror with Hunting Pattern

Warring States Period

Copper

Diameter 10.4 cm

三弦纽，方纽座。以双线勾连雷纹为地纹，双线内填碎点纹。地纹之上，双武士与双豹相间排列，作搏斗状。此镜虽出土于秦墓，实为战国遗物。1957 年湖北云梦睡虎地出土。

中国国家博物馆藏

The mirror has a three-string knob and a square knob pedestal. The two-string thunder pattern serves as the ground-tint pattern, and within the two steaks are the decorations of spot pattern. Upon the decorative pattern, there are two warriors together with two leopards which are alternately arranged. The warriors are fighting against the leopards. Although this mirror was unearthed from the tomb of Qin State, it actually belongs to the remains of Warring States Period. It was unearthed from Shuihudi, Yunmeng County, Hubei Province, in 1957.

Preserved in National Museum of China

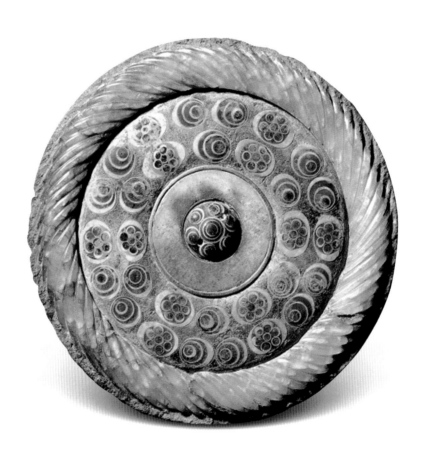

镶嵌玉琉璃镜

战国

琉璃

径 12.2 厘米

蓝色琉璃纽，间以白色套圈纹，以玉环为纽座。其外嵌六出花形与白色套圈相间的蓝色琉璃。镜缘为绳纹玉环。此镜做工独特，色彩艳丽，颇为珍贵。传洛阳金村出土。

哈佛艺术博物馆藏

Glazed Mirror Inlaid with Jade

Warring States Period

Glaze

Diameter 12.2 cm

The mirror has a blue glazed knob whose central part is decorated with white ferrule pattern. The pedestal of the knob is a jade ring. Outside the knob is the decoration of blue glaze which is the combination of six petals flower pattern and white ferrule pattern. The edge of the mirror is composed of jade rings with rope pattern. This mirror is uniquely designed with magnificent color and it's very precious. It is said that this mirror was unearthed from Jin Village of Luoyang City.

Preserved in Harvard Art Museums

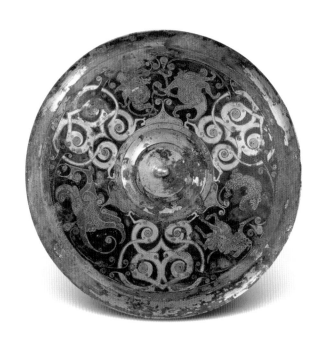

错金银狩猎纹镜

战国

铜质

径 17.5 厘米

Golden and Sliver Smeared Mirror with Hunting Pattern

Warring States Period

Copper

Diameter 17.5 cm

圆纽，圆纽座。镜背饰三组两两相对的连体龙纹，龙

纹间配置三组纹饰：一组为身披盔甲，持剑握缰的骑士，

欲刺一张牙舞爪的猛虎；一组为两兽搏斗；另一组为

一只展翅的凤鸟。纹饰皆错金丝，龙纹躯体并错银丝。

镜体为夹层，以镜背外缘包嵌镜面而成。传河南洛阳

金村出土。

日本永清文库藏

The mirror has a round knob with round pedestal. The
back part of the mirror is decorated with three groups of
dragon patterns which are alternately arranged in pairs.
The spare spaces among the dragon patterns are decorated
with three groups of different patters: the first one depicts
a knight who wears armor and holds sword and habena in
his hands, and ready to stab the fierce-looking tiger; the
second one depicts a scene that two animals fight against
each other; the third one is the decoration of a flying
phoenix. All the decorations are smeared with gold wires
and the body of the dragon is smeared with silver wires.
The mirror has an interlayer which is the combination of
the mirror face and the outer edge of its back side. It is
said that this mirror was unearthed from Jin Village of
Luoyang City.

Preserved in Yongqing Library, Japan

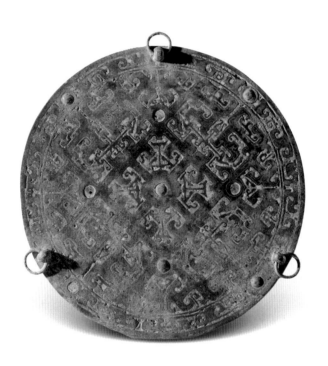

镶嵌几何纹三纽镜

战国

铜质

径 29.8 厘米

Three-knob Mirror with Geometry Pattern

Warring States Period

Copper

Diameter 29.8 cm

镜背饰四组几何纹，并以云纹为边框，整
个纹饰嵌金丝和绿松石，中间和边缘间嵌
银质乳钉九枚，镜缘均匀地饰三个环纽。
此镜形体硕大，色彩绚丽，为青铜镜中所
稀见。1963 年山东临淄齐国故城出土。

山东博物馆藏

The back side of the mirror is decorated with
four groups of geometry patterns and the
rim is decorated with cloud-like pattern. The
whole patterns are smeared with gold wire
and kallaite. The central part and the rim are
smeared with nine silver nails. The rim is
evenly decorated with three ring-like knobs.
This mirror is large in size and magnificent
in color, which is rarely seen among bronze
wares. It was unearthed from the ruins of Qi
State in Linzi City, Shandong Province in
1963.

Preserved in Shandong Museum

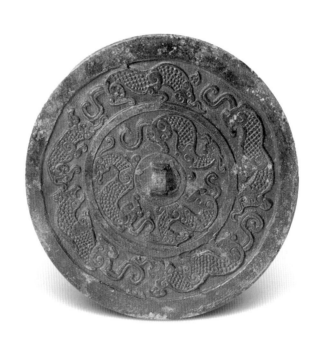

虎纹镜

战国

铜质

径 9.8 厘米

Mirror with Tiger Pattern

Warring States Period

Copper

Diameter 9.8 cm

桥形纽。内区饰三虎纹，皆回首卷尾；外区饰五虎纹，竖耳卷尾，作追逐状，其中一虎较小。1978 年陕西凤翔雍城出土。

凤翔县博物馆藏

The mirror has a bridge-shaped knob. The inside part is decorated with the pattern of three tigers and all the tigers turn their heads back and curl their tails up. On the outside part is decorative pattern of five tigers, which are chasing each other with ears pricking up and tails curling up. Among the five tigers, one is smaller. It was excavated from Yongcheng in Fengxiang County, Shaanxi Province in 1978.

Preserved in Fengxiang County Museum

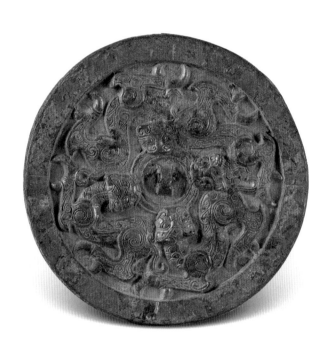

四虎纹镜

战国

铜质

径 12.1 厘米

Mirror with Four-tiger Pattern

Warring States Period

Copper

Diameter 12.1 cm

桥形纽，圆纽座。四虎作高浮雕，横置于
同一方向。虎头对着纽座，并用嘴咬住。
虎颈饰细毛，躯干饰雷纹。此镜具有三晋
地区铜镜风格。

上海博物馆藏

The mirror has a bridge-shaped knob whose
pedestal is round in shape. The four tigers
are placed horizontally towards the same
direction as high relief. The tigers are biting
the base of the knob with their heads toward
it. The neck of the tigers is decorated with
fine fur, while their bodies are adorned
with thunder pattern. The mirror has the
characteristics of bronze mirrors in ancient
Shanxi region (including three states: Han,
Zhao, and Wei in the Warring States Period).
Preserved in Shanghai Museum

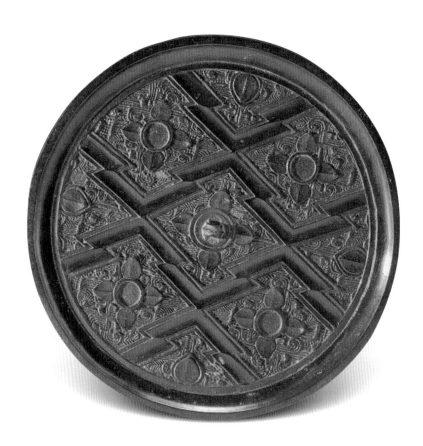

四瓣花菱纹镜

战国

铜质

径 11.8 厘米

三弦纽，圆纽座。以凹弧的曲折状菱纹将镜背分割成九小区，小区内饰四瓣花。地纹为深峻的羽状纹。1955 年湖南长沙廖家湾 38 号墓出土。

湖南省博物馆藏

Mirror with Lozenge Pattern with Quatrefoil

Warring States Period

Copper

Diameter 11.8 cm

The mirror has a three-string-shaped knob and round pedestal. The concave arc in bended lozenge pattern divides the back side of the mirror into nine sections, each of which is decorated with quatrefoil. The setoff pattern is deep feather-like pattern. It was excavated from No. 38 Tomb in Liaojiawan of Changsha City, Hunan Province in 1955.

Preserved in Hunan Museum

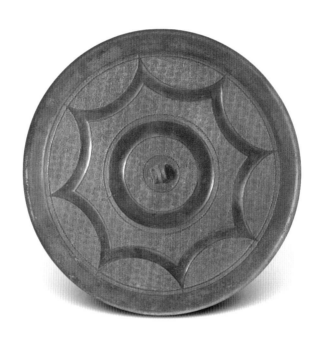

云雷纹地连弧纹铜镜

战国

铜质

直径 21.3 厘米

Bronze Mirror with Continuous Arc-like Patterns and Cloud-thunder as Setoff Patterns

Warring States Period

Bronze

Diameter 21.3 cm

Relics of Chinese Medicine and Health (First Series)
Metal　Volume Two　**329**

三弦纽，凹面形圆纽座。以一周绚纹将镜背分离为内区和外区。以云纹和三角形雷纹组成云雷地纹，主纹为八内向凹面连弧纹，弧纹的交点直达外缘。外区边缘有绚纹一周。宽素缘，低卷边，镜体较薄。战国中晚期楚国地区较为流行的铜镜。1993年扬州郊区西湖果园砖瓦厂战国木椁墓出土。

扬州博物馆藏

The mirror has a three-string-shaped knob and concave pedestal. A circle of intertwined rope-like pattern divides the backside of the mirror into inner section and outer section. It is decorated with setoff patterns of cloud and triangle thunder as well as eight inward concave continuous arc-like patterns as main ornaments. The intersections of arc-like patterns reach the outer edge of the mirror. The edge of the outer section has a circle of intertwined rope-like pattern. The body is thin with broad simple edge and low crimping. It was popular in Chu State in middle and late Warring States Period. The mirror was excavated from Timber Tomb of Warring States in Western Lake Orchard Bricks and Tiles Plant at Suburb of Yangzhou in 1993.

Preserved in Yangzhou Museum

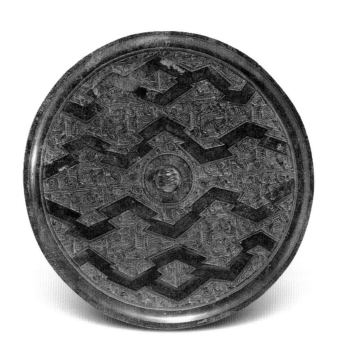

变形菱纹镜

战国

铜质

径 13 厘米

Mirror with Deformed Diamond Patterns

Warring States Period

Copper

Diameter 13 cm

三弦纽，圆纽座。主题纹饰为变形菱纹，呈凹弧曲折状，这是山字纹的一种变形；以羽状纹为地纹。1980 年湖南益阳赫山镇出土。

益阳市博物馆藏

The mirror has a three-string-shaped knob whose pedestal is round. Main decorative patterns are deformed diamond patterns, shaped like zigzag of concave arc, which is a transformation of patterns with Chinese character " 山 "(shan). The setoff patterns are feather-like. It was excavated from Heshan Town in Yiyang City of Hunan Province in 1980.

Preserved in Yiyang City Museum

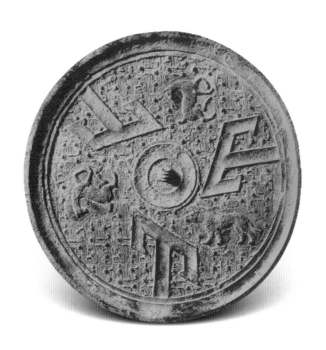

三山瑞兽纹镜

战国

铜质

径 20 厘米

Mirror with Auspicious Animal Pattern and Three Characters "Shan"

Warring States Period

Copper

Diameter 20 cm

四弦纽，圆纽座。主题纹饰是三山和三兽相间环列。一兽似犬，作前视状，竖耳垂尾；两兽似鹿，作回首屈肢状，形态生动。以羽纹为地纹。三山纹镜以三兽相间的仅见此镜。

巴黎博物馆藏

The mirror has a four-string-shaped knob whose pedestal is round. The main decorative patterns are three Chinese characters " 山 " (shan) alternated with three animals arranged in a circle. One of the animals is shaped like a dog looking forward with its ears upright and tail hanging down. The other two are deer with their heads turning back and limbs bending, which is very vivid. The setoff patterns are feather-like. In all mirrors with patterns of three characters " 山 " (shan), only this mirror is characterized with three alternated animals.

Preserved in Paris Museum

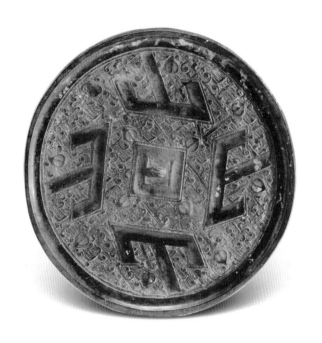

四山纹镜

战国

铜质

径 14.2 厘米

Mirror with Four Characters "Shan"

Warring States Period

Copper

Diameter 14.2 cm

三弦纽，方纽座。方框四角引出条带纹，上缀花瓣，四山形纹与带纹交叉重叠。地纹为深峻的羽状纹。1952 年湖南长沙燕山岭 855 号墓出土。

湖南省博物馆藏

The mirror has a three-string-shaped knob whose pedestal is square. Four corners of the square pedestal bring four ribbon-like patterns, which are decorated with petals as well as crossed and overlapped with the patterns of four Chinese characters " 山 " (shan). The mirror is adorned with setoff patterns of deep feather-like design. It was excavated from No. 855 Tomb in Yanshan Mountain, Changsha City, Hunan Province in 1952. Preserved in Hunan Museum

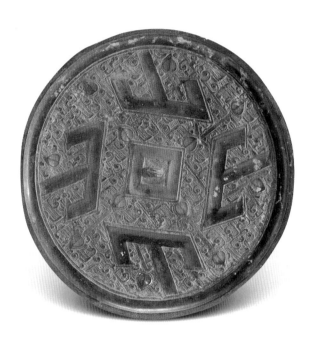

四山纹镜

战国

铜质

径 16.4 厘米

Mirror with Four Characters "Shan"

Warring States Period

Copper

Diameter 16.4 cm

三弦纽，方形纽座。主纹为四山纹，底边
与方纽座的每一边平行。纽座四角歧出的
花瓣，一枝作为四山纹的间隔，另一枝置
于四山纹的中间。纹饰的空隙处填以羽纹。

上海博物馆藏

The mirror has a three-string-shaped knob
whose pedestal is square. It is mainly
characterized by the pattern of four Chinese
characters " 山 "(shan) with each of their
bottoms parallel to one line of the square
pedestal. Among petals branching from four
corners of the square pedestal, one separates
the four characters " 山 " (shan), while the
other is located among those characters.
Spaces in the decorative patterns are filled
with feather-like patterns.

Preserved in Shanghai Museum

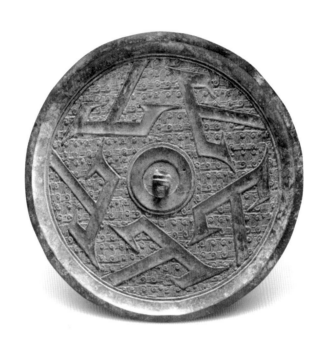

五山字纹铜镜

战国

铜质

直径 14.67 厘米

Copper Mirror with Five Characters "Shan"

Warring States Period

Copper

Diameter 14.67 cm

三弦纽，圆纽座。主题纹饰为五山纹，纹
饰的空隙处填以羽纹。

　　　　　　　湖北省文物考古研究所藏

The mirror has a three-string-shaped knob
whose pedestal is round. It is mainly
characterized by the pattern of five Chinese
characters " 山 " (shan). Spaces in the
decorative patterns are filled with feather-
like pattern.
Preserved in Institute of Cultural Relics and
Archaeology of Hubei Province

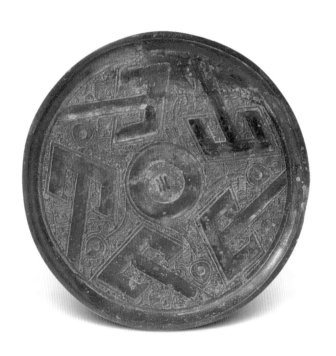

五山纹铜镜

战国

铜质

直径 16 厘米

Copper Mirror with Five Characters "Shan"

Warring States Period

Copper

Diameter 16 cm

三弦纽，圆纽座，主题纹饰为五山纹和纽座引出的缀有花瓣的条状纹。地纹为羽纹。战国早期的铜镜小而薄，后来趋向稍大而厚重，题材以蟠螭纹和云雷纹最流行，加上粗线条的山字纹的镜最具有代表性。

梁就藏

The mirror has a three-string-shaped knob whose pedestal is round. It is mainly characterized by the pattern of five Chinese characters " 山 " (shan) and ribbon-like patterns bringing from the pedestal, which are decorated with petals. The mirror is adorned with the patterns of feather-like design. Mirrors in early Warring States Period is small and thin, but later tend to be big and heavy. Among the decorative patterns, Pan Chi (a kind of dragons without horns in ancient Chinese legends) pattern and cloud and thunder patterns were most popular and the most representative mirrors are decorated with those patterns as well as inscribed with bolded Chinese character " 山 " (shan).

Collected by Liang Jiu

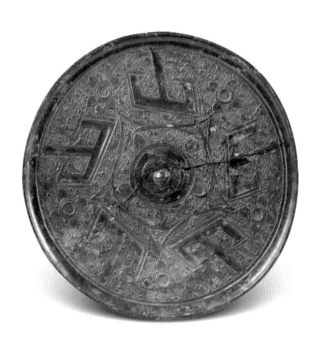

五山纹镜

战国

铜质

直径 16.5 厘米

Mirror with Five Characters "Shan"

Warring States Period

Copper

Diameter 16.5 cm

单弦纽，圆纽座。纽座外五出花瓣纹，外围由宽弧线组成重叠五瓣花形似五角星纹，星角对应一圆心四瓣花朵，花朵间逆时针排列五个山字，底边与星边相对。以羽状纹为地纹。

中国国家博物馆藏

The mirror has a single-string-shaped knob whose pedestal is round. Five petals pattern decorates the external of the pedestal. Surrounding the five petals pattern is an overlapping pentagram-like flower of five petals, which is shaped by a broad arc. Each angle of the pentagram corresponds to a quatrefoil with a ring-like center. Among the quatrefoil are anticlockwise arranged five characters of " 山 " (shan). The bottoms of those characters are opposing to the lines of the pentagram and are decorated with feather-like setoff patterns.

Preserved in National Museum of China

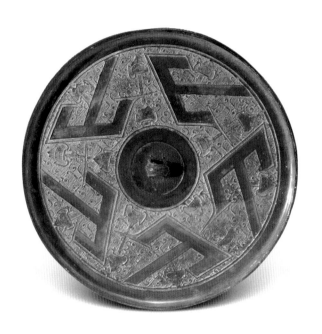

五山纹镜

战国

铜质

径 18.8 厘米

Mirror with Five Characters "Shan"

Warring States Period

Copper

Diameter 18.8 cm

四弦纽，圆纽座。由圆座外圈引出五条带纹，上各缀二枫叶状花瓣，五山字纹右旋。地纹为深峻羽状纹。1958 年湖南常德德山出土。

湖南省博物馆藏

The mirror has a four-string-shaped knob whose pedestal is round. The outer ring of the round pedestal brings five ribbon-like patterns, and each of them is decorated with two maple leaf-like petals. The pattern of five Chinese characters "山" (shan) rotates to the right side. The mirror is decorated with deep feather-like setoff patterns and was excavated from Deshan Mountain in Changde City of Hunan Province, in 1958.

Preserved in Hunan Museum

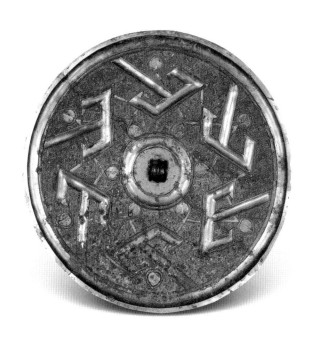

六山纹镜

战国

铜质

直径 23.2 厘米

Mirror with Six Characters "Shan"

Warring States Period

Copper

Diameter 23.2 cm

三弦纽，圆纽座。主纹为逆时针排列六山字，山字修长，倾斜度较大，山字底边与相邻山字边的延长线相接，形成一六角星芒形。纽座外及山字上各饰小花瓣六个，均以羽状纹为地。此镜体形较大，纹饰精美。

中国国家博物馆藏

The mirror has a three-string-shaped knob whose pedestal is round. The main pattern is anticlockwise arranged six Chinese characters of " 山 " (shan) that are slender and incline to a large extent. The bottom line of " 山 " (shan) is connected with the extended line of one stroke of the adjacent character " 山 " (shan), forming a hexagram-like pattern. Six little petals are decorated on the outer pedestal and the characters of " 山 " (shan) respectively. The mirror takes feather-like patterns as setoff patterns. It is large, with exquisite decorative patterns.

Preserved in National Museum of China

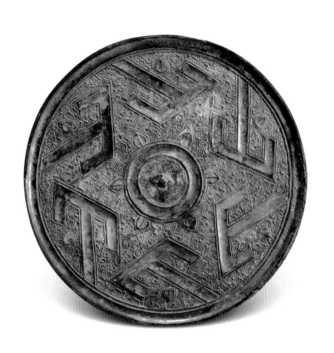

六山纹镜

战国

铜质

径 21.2 厘米

Mirror with Six Characters "Shan"

Warring States Period

Copper

Diameter 21.2 cm

三弦纽，圆纽座。连续排成一周的山字纹甚倾斜，纽座旁有六叶，填于山字之间的空隙，每一山字上又有一叶作装饰。六山纹镜较为罕见。1983 年广东广州象岗山南越王墓出土。

西汉南越王博物馆藏

The mirror has a three-string-shaped knob whose pedestal is round. The pattern is quite gradient with six Chinese characters " 山 " (shan) continuously arranged in a circle. Beside the pedestal are six leafs, filling the spaces among the characters of " 山 " (shan) and each character is decorated with a leaf. The mirror inscribed with six characters " 山 " (shan) is rare. It was excavated from Mausoleum of the Nanyue King in Xianggang Mountain of Guangzhou, Guangdong Province in 1983. Preserved in Museum of the Western Han Dynasty Mausoleum of the Nanyue King

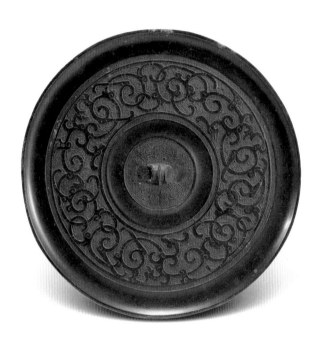

蟠龙纹镜

战国

铜质

直径 14.3 厘米

Copper Mirror with Curled-up Dragon Pattern

Warring States Period

Copper

Diameter 14.3 cm

三弦纽，圆纽座。主题纹饰为盘曲的三龙，

龙身缠绕如枝蔓，以细密的云纹为地纹。

1955 年湖南长沙燕子嘴 17 号墓出土。

湖南省博物馆藏

The mirror has a three-string-shaped knob
whose pedestal is round. The mirror is mainly
decorated with three intertwined dragons
with their bodies twined like branches,
taking elaborated cloud as setoff patterns. It
was excavated from No. 17 Yanzizui Tomb in
Changsha City of Hunan Province in 1955.
Preserved in Hunan Museum

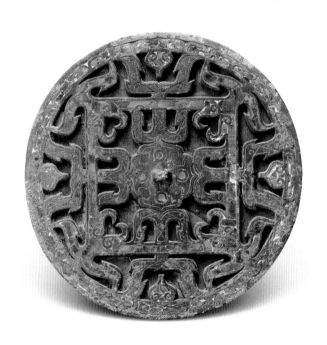

镶嵌绿松石透雕几何纹镜

战国

铜质

直径 10.6 厘米

Mirror with Openwork Geometric Pattern and Inlaid Kallaite

Warring States Period

Copper

Diameter 10.6 cm

小纽，四瓣莲花纹纽座。内区呈方形，沿纽座饰花纹。方框以外为外区，四方各饰几何形图案，图案上有纤细的云纹。纽座、方框及镜缘外都用绿松石镶嵌。

日本千石唯司藏

The mirror has a little knob whose pedestal is decorated with lotus of four petals pattern. Inside part of the mirror is square, and the decorative pattern is along the pedestal. Outside the square is the outer part, which is decorated with geometric patterns with fine cloud patterns on it. Kallaite are inlaid into the pedestal of the knob, the square and the outer edge of the mirror.

Preserved by Sengoku Yuishi, Japan

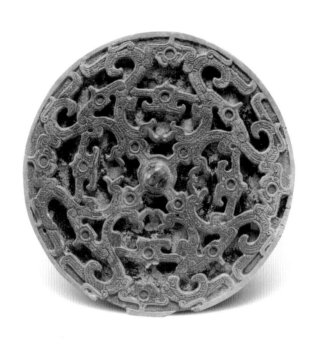

镂空凤纹铜镜

战国

铜质

直径 11 厘米

Copper Mirror with Hollowed-out Phoenix Pattern

Warring States Period

Copper

Diameter 11 cm

圆形小纽，以十字将纹饰分为四部分，每部分镂雕凤鸟一对，头相对，身体弯曲，尾部向外翻翘。空隙处以卷云纹相连。1985 年湖北省荆州市江陵酒店 315 号墓出土。

湖北省博物馆藏

The patterns on the mirror are divided into four parts by small round knobs. Each part has a couple of hollowed-out engraved opposite phoenixes with bent bodies and warped tails. Spaces in the decorative patterns are filled with cloud-like patterns. It was unearthed from No. 315 Jiangling Hotel Tomb in Jingzhou City of Hubei Province in 1985.

Preserved in Hubei Provincial Museum

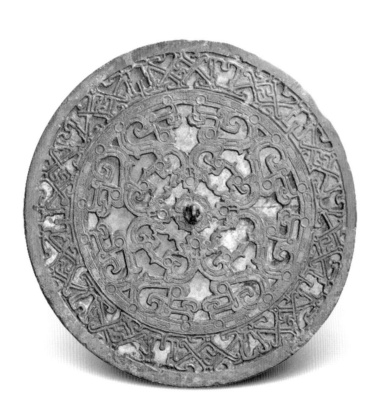

透雕龙凤纹镜

战国

铜质

直径 20.5 厘米

透雕圆纽，柿蒂纹纽座。镜双层结合，镜背嵌入镜面。一周云雷纹将纹饰分为内、外两区，内区是透雕蜷曲的龙凤纹四组；外区饰双线交叉几何纹，缘平素无纹。此镜纹饰精美，工艺精细。1976 年湖北江陵张家山出土。

中国国家博物馆藏

Mirror with Openwork Dragon-phoenix Pattern

Warring States Period

Copper

Diameter 20.5 cm

The mirror has an openwork round knob whose pedestal is decorated with kaki calyx pattern. It has two connected layers, of which the rear of mirror embeds in the mirror face. A circle of cloud-thunder patterns divides the decorative patterns into two parts. The inside part is decorated with four groups of openwork curling up dragon-phoenix patterns. The outer section is adorned with geographic patterns of cross double lines. The edge is simple without patterns. The mirror is characterized by exquisite patterns and delicate craft. It was unearthed from Zhangjia Mountain, Jiangling County, Hubei Province in 1976.

Preserved in National Museum of China

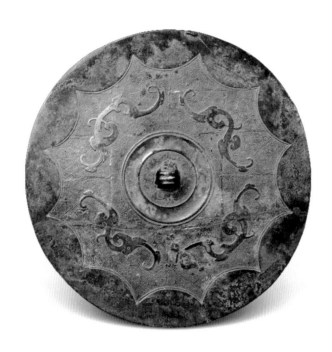

四凤纹镜

战国

铜质

直径 13.7 厘米

Mirror with Four-phoenix Pattern

Warring States Period

Copper

Diameter 13.7 cm

三弦纽，圆纽座。主题纹饰为四凤鸟环纽

配列，地纹为云雷纹，边缘饰连弧纹。

1957 年陕西西安郊区出土。

陕西历史博物馆藏

The mirror has a three-string-like knob
whose pedestal is round. The main decorative
pattern is that of four phoenixes arranged
around the knob with cloud-thunder patterns
as setoff patterns. The edge is decorated with
continuous arc-like patterns. It was excavated
from suburb of Xi'an, Shaanxi Province in
1957.

Preserved in Shaanxi History Museum

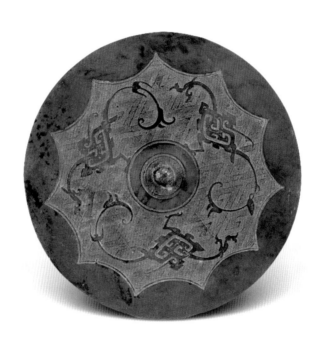

三龙纹镜

战国

铜质

直径 15.9 厘米

Mirror with Three-dragon Pattern

Warring States Period

Copper

Diameter 15.9 cm

双弦纽，圆纽座。主题纹饰为三龙纹，龙长尾，一足而立，作追逐状；以云纹组成的勾连雷纹为地纹，边缘饰十一个内向连弧纹。1975 年安徽和县西汉墓出土。

安徽博物院藏

The mirror has a two-string-like knob whose pedestal is round. The main decorative pattern is that of three dragons with long tails and one standing foot chasing with each other. The setoff pattern is connected with thunder pattern set off by cloud patterns. The edge is decorated with eleven inward continuous arc-like patterns. It was excavated from the Tomb of Western Han Dynasty in Hexian County, Anhui Province in 1975. Preserved in Anhui Museum

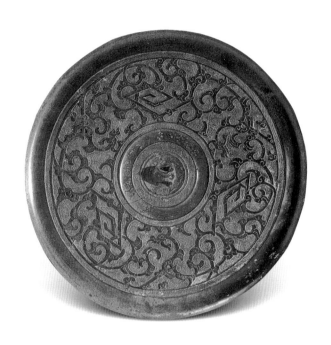

三龙纹镜

战国

铜质

直径 15.2 厘米

Mirror with Three-dragon Pattern

Warring States Period

Copper

Diameter 15.2 cm

四弦纽，圆纽座。主题纹饰为三组变形龙纹，龙身盘曲如枝蔓，龙与龙之间相交接处饰勾连菱形图案。1952 年湖南长沙蓉园 856 号墓出土。

湖南省博物馆藏

The mirror has a four-string-like knob whose pedestal is round. The main decorative pattern is three groups of morphed dragons with their bodies twined like branches. Where the dragons intersect is decorated with connected diamond-like patterns. It was excavated from No. 856 Rongyuan Tomb of Changsha City, Hunan Province in 1952. Preserved in Hunan Museum

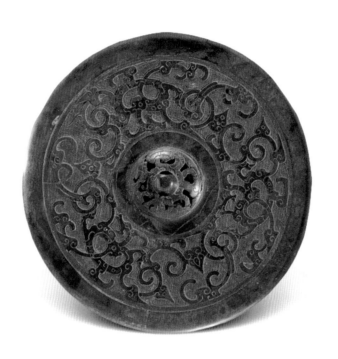

三龙纹镂空纽镜

战国

铜质

直径 16.5 厘米

Mirror with Three-dragon Pattern and Hollowed-out Knob

Warring States Period

Copper

Diameter 16.5 cm

镂空圆纽。主纹为三龙，龙身如蔓枝，极具图案化，龙首有独角，张口露齿；地纹为细密的云雷纹。1953 年湖南长沙子弹库出土。

湖南省博物馆藏

The mirror has a hollowed-out knob. The main decorative pattern is three dragons with their bodies twined like branches, which look quite pictorialized. There is a horn on the head of the dragon that is opening its mouth and showing its teeth. The setoff patterns are exquisite cloud and thunder patterns. The mirror was excavated from Zidanku in Changsha City of Hunan Province in 1953. Preserved in Hunan Museum

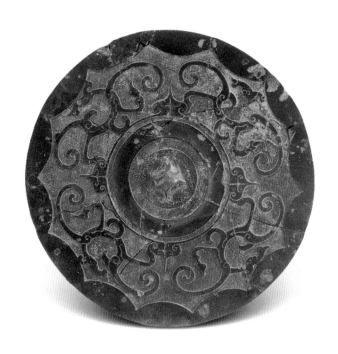

四龙纹镜

战国

铜质

直径 14.5 厘米

Mirror with Four-dragon Pattern

Warring States Period

Copper

Diameter 14.5 cm

三弦纽，圆纽座。主题纹饰为四条盘曲的
龙，张口卷尾，线条简洁，间以莲瓣状叶
纹。以细密的雷纹、三角纹为地纹。边缘
饰十四个内向连弧纹。1955 年湖南长沙
潘家坪 6 号墓出土。

湖南省博物馆藏

The mirror has a three-string-like knob
whose pedestal is round. The main decorative
pattern is four dragons with their bodies
intertwined, mouths opening and tails curling
up. The dragons have succinct lines and are
separated by lotus petal-like leaf patterns.
The setoff patterns are exquisite thunder
patterns and triangle patterns. The edge is
decorated with fourteen inward continuous
arc-like patterns. It was excavated from No.6
Panjiaping Tomb in Changsha City of Hunan
Province in 1955.

Preserved in Hunan Museum

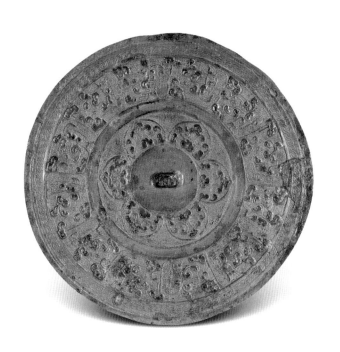

变形龙纹镜

战国

铜质

直径 11 厘米

Mirror with Deformed Dragon Pattern

Warring States Period

Copper

Diameter 11 cm

桥形纽。内区为六片莲瓣纹，内饰羽翅状
龙纹，外区环列十二组变形龙纹，边缘饰
绚纹一周。1965 年山西长治出土。

山西博物院藏

The knob of the mirror is shaped like a
bridge. The inside part is decorated with
six lotus petal patterns, in which there is
wing-like dragon pattern. The outside part
is circulated by twelve groups of deformed
dragon patterns and the edge is decorated
with a circle of intertwined rope-like pattern.
It was excavated from Changzhi City in
Shanxi Province in 1965.
Preserved in Shanxi Museum

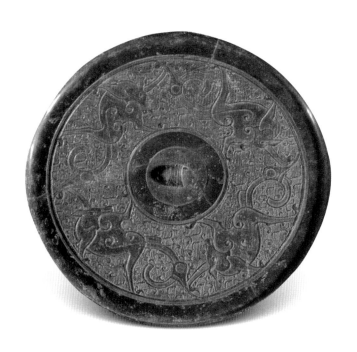

四兽纹彩绘镜

战国

铜质

直径 19 厘米

Colored-drawing Mirror with Four-animal Pattern

Warring States Period

Copper

Diameter 19 cm

三弦纽，圆纽座。主题纹饰为四兽，兽身扭转，张口竖耳，兽尾极长，尾端似有一花结。以羽状纹为地纹。镜缘朱绘菱纹，大部已脱落。1952 年湖南长沙斗笠坡 744 号墓出土。

湖南省博物馆藏

The mirror has a three-string-like knob whose pedestal is round. The main decorative pattern is four mythical creatures (azure dragon, white tiger, rosefinch, and tortoise) with their bodies turning round, ears pricking up and mouths opening. Those creatures have very long tails which seem to have knots at the end of them. Feather-like patterns are used as setoff patterns. The edge of the mirror is painted with red diamond-like patterns, but most of them had come off. It was excavated from No. 744 Doulipo Tomb in Changsha City of Hunan Province in 1952. Preserved in Hunan Museum

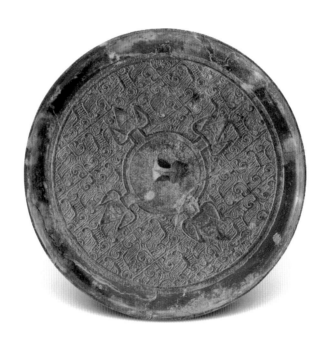

四叶纹镜

战国

铜质

直径 11.7 厘米

Mirror with Four-leaf Pattern

Warring States Period

Copper

Diameter 11.7 cm

三弦纽，圆纽座。主题纹饰为四叶纹，均匀地排列在纽座外的弦纹上，叶外以羽状纹和细点纹为地。1952 年湖南长沙丝茅冲 78 号墓出土。

湖南省博物馆藏

The mirror has a three-string-like knob whose pedestal is round. It is mainly decorated with four leaf pattern, which is evenly arranged on the string patterns outside the knob pedestal. Feather-like and fine-point patterns are decorated outside the leaves as setoff patterns. It was excavated from No.78 Simaochong Tomb in Changsha City of Hunan Province in 1952.

Preserved in Hunan Museum

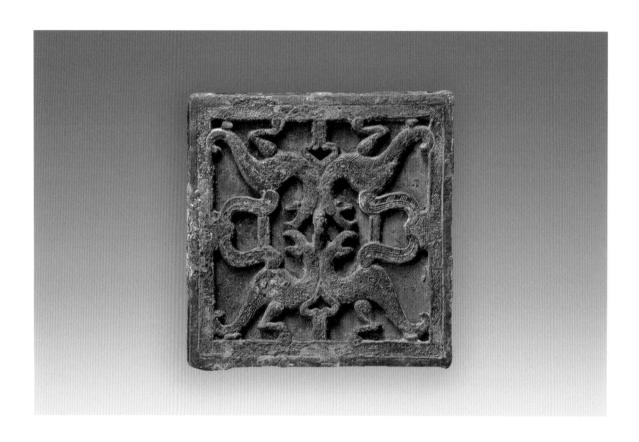

透雕凤纹方镜

战国

铜质

边长 8 厘米

Square Mirror with Openwork Phoenix Pattern

Warring States Period

Copper

Length 8 cm

镂空圆纽。主纹为四凤，凤呈侧面，长颈回顾，躬背、卷尾，腹下仅见一足，两凤颈部相接作对称状排列，凤头顶与另三组凤纹相接，构成四方图案，四凤的颈部连接一小环成为纽座。边框及所有纹饰上都有很细的线条和三角纹。此镜除氧化层外还留有朱砂痕迹，使镜背纹饰增加了色彩。

日本千石唯司藏

The mirror has a hollowed-out round knob. It is mainly decorated with four-phoenix pattern, which depicts a side view of the phoenixes that look back. The phoenixes have long neck, bowed back, coiled tail and only one foot under the belly. Two phoenixes are connected by their necks, and arranged in symmetrical way. Their heads are connected, forming a square and necks are connected by a small ring, constituting the pedestal of the knob. On the rim and all of the patterns are slender lines and triangle patterns. Besides the oxide layer, there is vestige of cinnabar, which makes the patterns on the rear of the mirror more colorful.

Preserved by Sengoku Yuishi, Japan

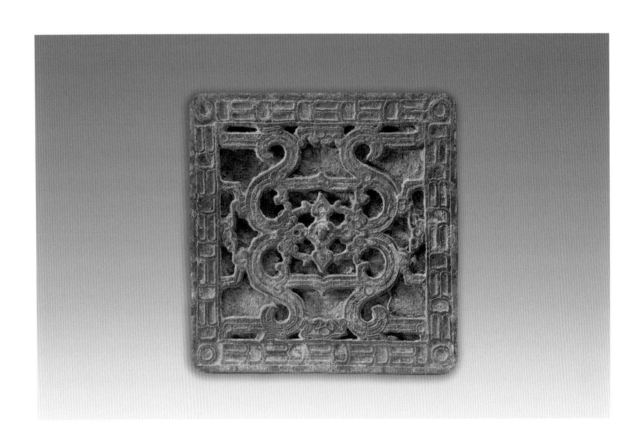

透雕龙纹方镜

战国

铜质

长 11.2 厘米，宽 11 厘米

Square Mirror with Openwork Dragon Pattern

Warring States Period

Copper

Length 11.2 cm/ Width 11 cm

半环形纽，柿蒂纽座。内区为两个相对的透雕回首卷龙纹，外区为重环纹。方形透雕镜在战国时期较为罕见。1988 年河南洛阳西工区出土。

洛阳博物馆藏

The mirror has a half ring-like knob whose pedestal is shaped like kaki calyx. The inside part is decorated with openwork of two opposing rolling dragon patterns and the outside part is multiple ring-like pattern. Square mirror with openwork sculpture is rare in the Warring States Period. It was excavated from Xigong District of Luoyang City in Henan Province in 1988.

Preserved in Luoyang Museum

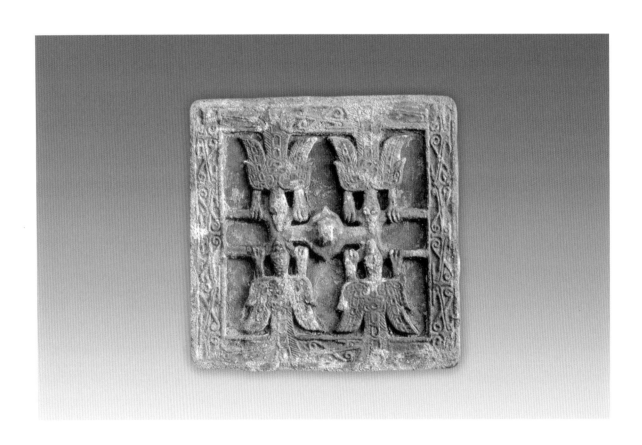

透雕四鸟纹方镜

战国

铜质

边长 8 厘米

Square Mirror with Openwork Four-bird Pattern

Warring States Period

Copper

Length 8 cm

镜背中间有一横档，上有小纽，叶形纽座，横档各分二枝与镜边相接。主纹为鸟，呈背向展翅状，伸出二爪攀附于横枝上。鸟体、羽翼各有羽毛纹，其间用朱砂填色，四边饰云纹。

日本千石唯司藏

At the center of the rear of the mirror is a horizontal beam with a little knob whose pedestal is shaped like a leaf. Both ends of the horizontal beam divide into two branches connected with the edge. The mirror is mainly decorated with birds, which are spreading their wings and stretching out the claws to climb on the horizontal beam. The bodies and wrings of the birds are decorated with feather-like patterns. Cinnabar is used to fill the space of the feather-like patterns. Four edges are decorated with cloud patterns. Preserved by Sengoku Yuishi, Japan

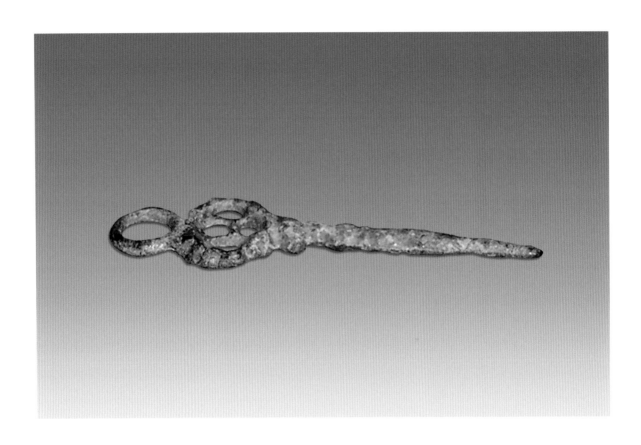

铜笄

战国

铜质

长 6 厘米，宽 1.5 厘米，重 1 千克

Copper Pin

Warring States Period

Copper

Length 6 cm/ Width 1.5 cm/ Weight 1 kg

头呈尖锥形，把呈双环状。发叉，生活用器。

完整无损。内蒙古征集。

陕西医史博物馆藏

The head is awl-like and the handle is made of two rings. It is an intact hairpin, belonging to life utensil. This copper pin was collected from Inner Mongolia.

Preserved in Shaanxi Museum of Medical History

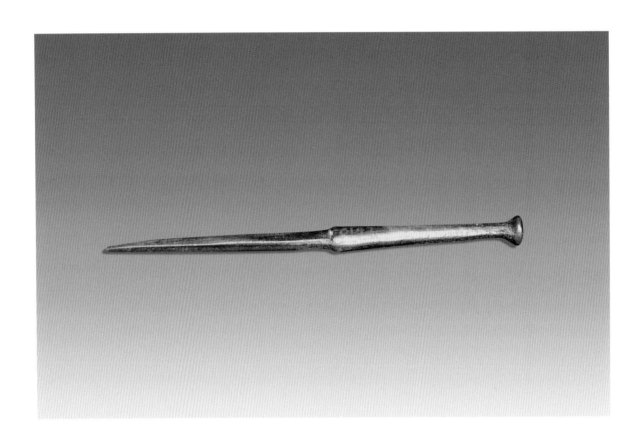

铜锥

战国

铜质

长 10.4 厘米，重 0.012 千克

Copper Awl

Warring States Period

Copper

Length 10 cm/ Weight 0.012 kg

锥头呈三棱形，锥把呈圆形。生活用具。

完整无损。内蒙古自治区东胜征集。

陕西医史博物馆藏

The head is tri-prism-like and the handle is round. This intact bronze awl belongs to life utensil and was collected from Dongsheng in the Inner Mongolia Autonomous Region.

Preserved in Shaanxi Museum of Medical History

错金银鸟纹虎子

战国后期

铜质

宽 22.6 厘米，底径 12.4 厘米，通高 13.6 厘米，重 1.7 千克

"Huzi" with Bird Pattern Smeared with Gold and Sliver

Late Warring States Period

Copper

Width 22.6 cm/ Bottom Diameter 13.6 cm/ Height 13.6 cm/ Weight 1.7 kg

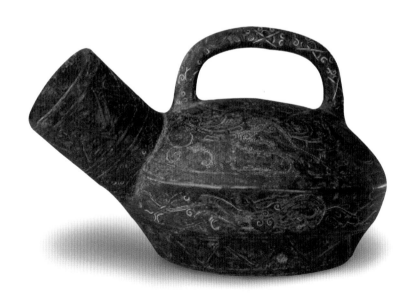

器扁圆，大腹，有流，有鋬。通体饰金银丝镶嵌纹饰，腹部以鸟纹为主题纹饰，口部、腹下饰 V 形连纹，底部饰嵌金涡纹。虎子为溺器。1954 年收购。

故宫博物院藏

The vessel is flattened circular with a large belly, a spout and a handle. There is gold-silver-inlaid pattern on the whole body, bird pattern on the belly, continuous V-shape patterns on the spout and the belly as well as gold vortex pattern on the base. "Huzi" is a urine vessel and was collected in 1954.

Preserved in The Palace Museum

铲

战国前期

铜质

长 33.5 厘米，宽 23.3 厘米，重 1.5 千克

Shovel

Early Warring States Period

Copper

Length 33.5 cm/ Width 23.3 cm/ Weight 1.5 kg

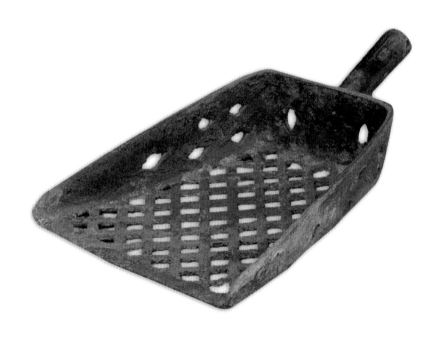

铜铲，柄中空，铲体呈网状镂空。1954
年收购。

故宫博物院藏

It is a bronze shovel with a hollow handle
and the body is like a hollowed-out net. The
shovel was acquired in 1954.
Preserved in The Palace Museum

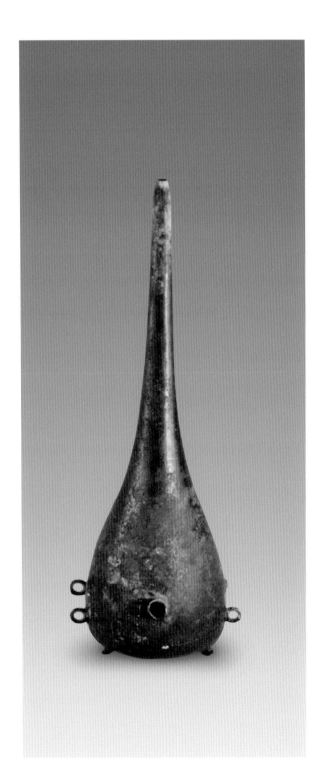

铜香熏

战国

铜质

盘口径 14 厘米，通高 42.8 厘米，重 2 千克

Copper Aromatherapy Heater

Warring States Period

Copper

Mouth Diameter of Plate 33.5 cm/ Height 42.8 cm/

Weigth 2 kg

用于燃熏香料、香草以散发香味。1978
年湖北随州市曾侯乙墓出土。

湖北省博物馆藏

The vessel was used for aromatic fumigation.
It was unearthed in Zeng Marquis Yi Tomb
of Warring States of Suizhou City, Hubei
Province, in 1978.
Preserved in Hubei Provincial Museum

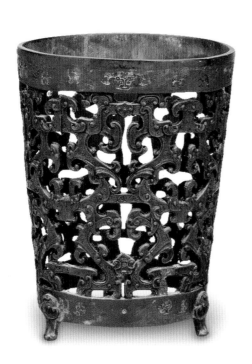

凤纹铜熏

战国

铜质

口径 14.3 厘米，通高 7.5 厘米

Aromatherapy Heater with Phoenix Pattern

Warring States Period

Copper

Mouth Diameter 14.3 cm/ Height 7.5 cm

镂空凤纹，三足，用于燃熏香料、香草以
散发香味。1978 年湖北随州市曾侯乙墓
出土。

湖北省博物馆藏

This three-footed vessel, engraved into hollow
phoenix pattern, was used for aromatic
fumigation. It was unearthed in Zeng Marquis
Yi Tomb of Warring States of Suizhou City,
Hubei Province, in 1978.

Preserved in Hubei Provincial Museum

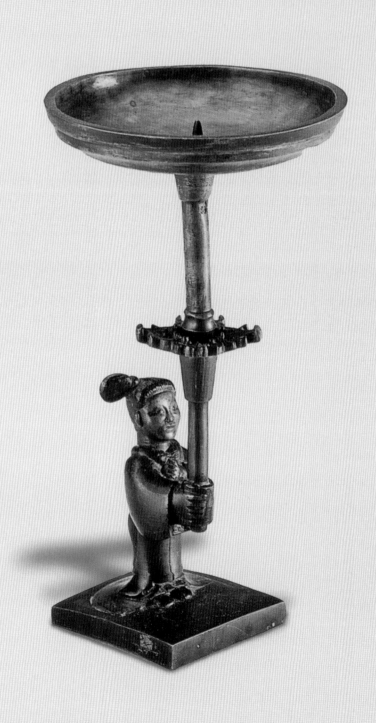

人擎铜灯

战国

铜质

通高 16.3 厘米

灯盘：口径 8.8 厘米

铜人：高 6.9 厘米

由灯盘和铜人两部分组成。灯盘较浅，直口，平沿，盘中有高 1 厘米的圆锥状灯纤。铜人头挽右髻，发髹黑漆，宽额，浓眉大眼，圆颔，耳微外侈，右衽，广袖。1987 年湖北省荆门包山 2 号墓出土。

湖北省博物馆藏

Copper Lamp Held-up by a Man

Warring States Period

Copper

Height 16.3 cm

Lamp Dish: Mouth Diameter 8.8 cm

Bronze Man: Height 6.9 cm

The lamp is composed of a lamp dish and a bronze man. The shallow lamp dish has a straight mouth and flat edge with a 1 cm conical wick on it. The bronze man has black hair, broad forehead, big eyes, heavy eyebrows, round jaw, full sleeves and folds his clothes to the right. It was unearthed from No. 2 Baoshan Tomb in Jingmen City of Hubei Province in 1987.

Preserved in Hubei Provincial Museum

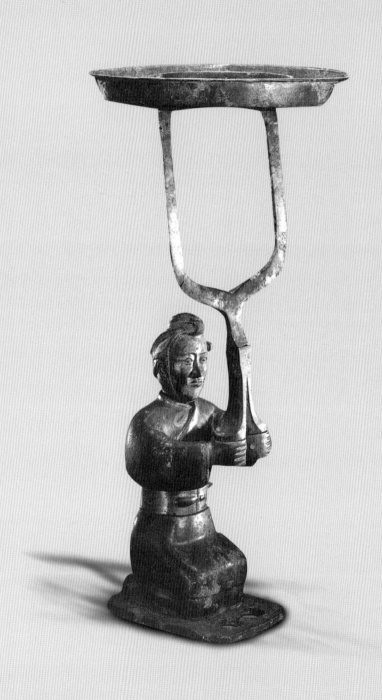

跽坐人漆绘灯

战国

铜质

通高 48.9 厘米

盘：径 23.7 厘米

由灯盘、灯架和跽坐人三部分组成。灯盘呈环形，内有三个烛座。灯架呈"丫"字形，其上连接灯盘，下端插入跽坐人手中。通体原髹黑漆，现已脱落。这件铜灯分为三部分，可进行拆装，且部件之间对接紧密。人物发式、服饰刻画入微。1975 年河南省三门峡上村岭出土。

河南博物院藏

Copper Kneeling Person-shaped Lamp

Warring States Period

Copper

Height 48.9 cm

Lamp Dish: Diameter 23.7 cm

The lamp is composed of a lamp dish, a lamp stand and a kneeling person. Three candlesticks are laid in the ring-like lamp dish. The kneeling person holds the fork-shaped lamp stand, the top of which is connected with the lamp dish. The surface of the lamp was painted by black paint but had come off. Three parts of the lamp are removable and the joint between each part is tight. The hair style and clothes of the person is quite exquisite. The lamp was excavated from Shangcunling in Sanmenxia City of Henan Province in 1975.

Preserved in Henan Museum

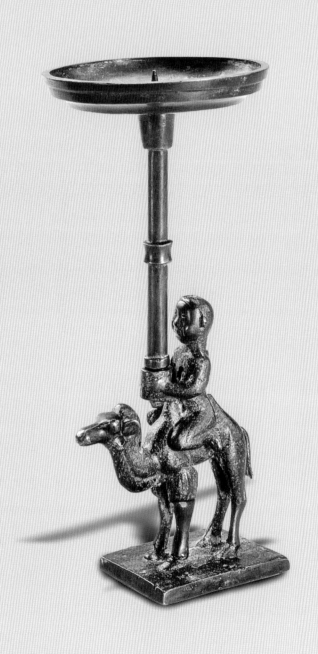

人骑骆驼铜灯

战国

铜质

通高 19.2 厘米

盘：径 8.8 厘米

柄：长 9.8 厘米

照明用具。由底座、骆驼、人物与灯柱、灯盘组成。长方形底座上立一人端坐驼身，手持圆形灯盘的灯柱。1965 年湖北江陵望山 2 号墓出土。

湖北省博物馆藏

Copper Lamp in the Shape of a Man Riding a Camel

Warring States Period

Copper

Height 19.2 cm

Dish: Diameter 8.8 cm

Handle: Length 9.8 cm

The lamp is utilized as a luminaire. It is composed of a pedestal, a camel, a figure, a lamp dish and a handle. The camel stands on the oblong pedestal with the figure sitting on it, holding the handle of the round lamp dish. It was unearthed from No. 2 Wangshan Tomb in Jiangling City of Hubei Province in 1965.

Preserved in Hubei Provincial Museum

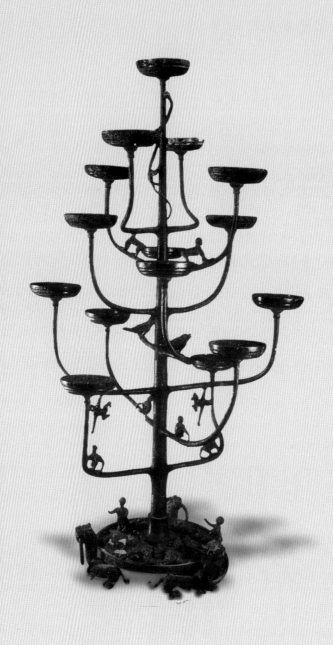

十五连盏灯

战国中期

铜质

宽 47 厘米，高 84.5 厘米

全灯形如茂盛的大树，由长短不同的八节接插而成，计十五个灯盘。镂孔透雕的圆形灯座，由三只一首二身、口衔环的虎承托。座上站立两个上身赤裸，下围短裙，手捧食物向上作抛食状的家奴。树上群猴戏耍，雀鸟鸣叫。树干顶上一蟠龙攀附。照明器具。

河北博物院藏

Lamp with 15 Disks

Mid Warring States Period

Copper

Width 47 cm/ Height 84.5 cm

The lamp is similar to a frondent tree, composing of 15 lamp disks on 8 branches different in length. The round pedestal is designed in hollow engraving pattern, held by three tiger-shaped sculptures. Each tiger has one head and two bodies, with a ring in mouth. There are two slave-shaped sculptures standing above the pedestal. The two slaves are throwing food away, topless with short skirts. On the tree, there are monkeys playing and birds singing. There is a dragon climbing on the top of the tree. It is utilized as a luminaire.

Preserved in Hebei Museum

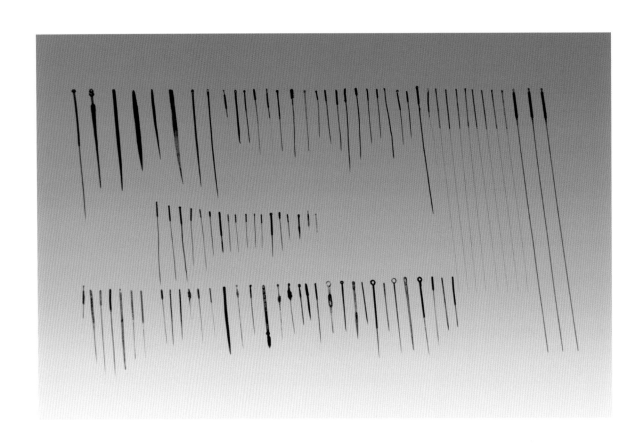

针灸针具

战国

金属

长 2.5 ~ 50 厘米

Acupuncture Needles

Warring States Period

Metal

Length 2.5–50 cm

共 91 枚，包括战国时期九针、火针、梅
花针、长针等。不同时期的针具具有不同
的特点，一般规律是随着时间的推移，针
灸针具越来越精致，越来越锋利。

北京御生堂中医药博物馆藏

There are 91 needles in this collection including
nine needles, fire needles, plum-blossom
needles and long needles from the Warring
States Period. The needles in different
periods of time have different features.
With time, the craftsmanship of needle-
making became more and more exquisite and
developed.

Preserved in Chinese Medicine Museum of
Beijing Yu Sheng Tang Drugstore

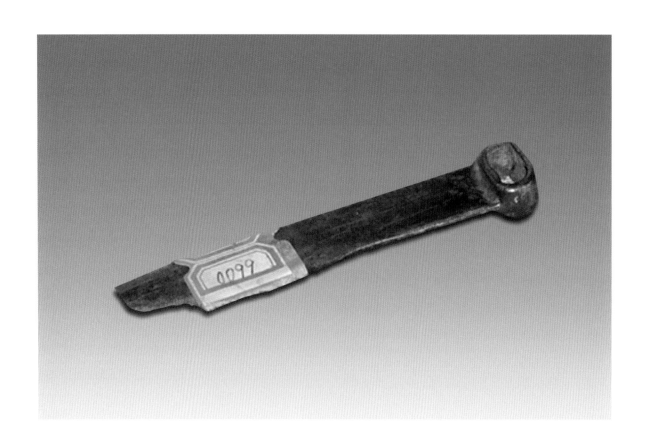

铜刀

战国

黄铜

长 10 厘米，宽 2 厘米，重 0.05 千克

Brass Broadsword

Warring States Period

Brass

Length 10 cm/ Width 2 cm/ Weight 0.05 kg

兵器。刀状，刀把处有一孔。刀尖残。内
蒙古自治区成陵征集。

陕西医史博物馆藏

The broadsword is a weapon. It is in the shape
of blade. There is a hole on the hilt and the
point of the blade is damaged. It was collected
from a Inner Mongolia Autonomous Region.
Preserved in Shaanxi Museum of Medical History

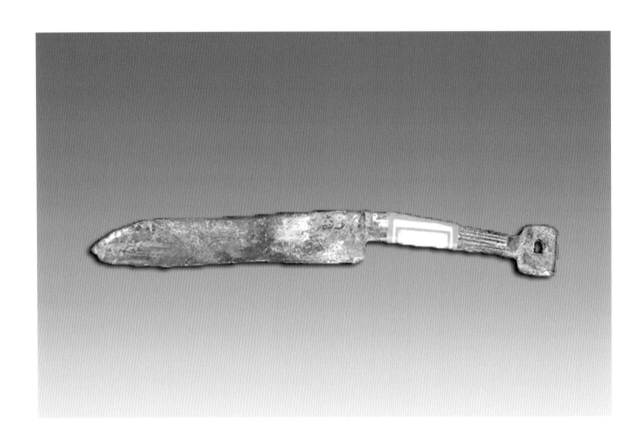

铜刀

战国

铜质

通长 17 厘米，重 0.06 千克

Copper Broadsword

Warring States Period

Copper

Length 17 cm/ Weight 0.06 kg

兵器。刀稍弯，刀把头呈方形，刀把有长
条纹。完整无损。陕西省西安市征集。

陕西医史博物馆藏

The broadsword is a weapon. The blade
curves slightly and the hilt is square shaped
with long stripes pattern. It is still in good
condition. It was collected from Xi'an,
Shaanxi Province.

Preserved in Shaanxi Museum of Medical History

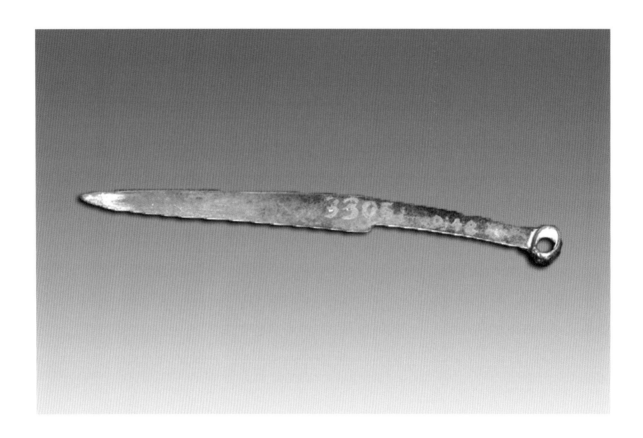

铜刀

战国

铜质

长 13.6 厘米，重 0.018 千克

Copper Broadsword

Warring States Period

Copper

Length 13.6 cm/ Weight 0.018 kg

兵器。刀稍弯，刀把扁平。完整无损。内
蒙古自治区东胜征集。

陕西医史博物馆藏

The broadsword is a weapon. The blade
curves slightly and the hilt is flat. It is still in
good condition. It was collected from Inner
Mongolia Autonomous Region.

Preserved in Shaanxi Museum of Medical History

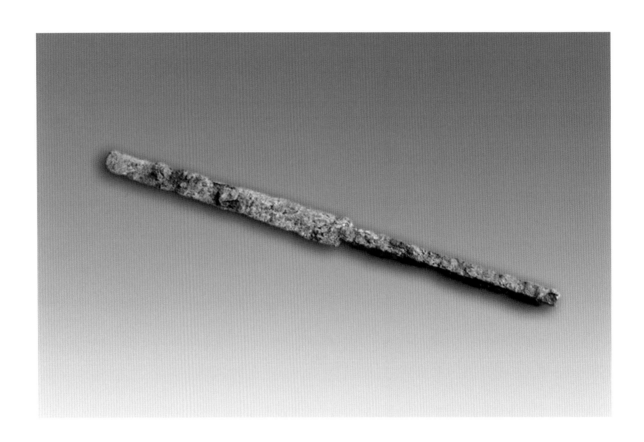

刀

战国

铁

长 42 厘米

Broadsword

Warring States Period

Iron

Length 42 cm

由成都市考古队调拨。

成都中医药大学中医药传统文化博物馆藏

The broadsword was allocated by Chengdu
Archaeological Team.

Preserved in Museum of Traditional Chinese
Medicine Culture, Chengdu University of
Traditional Chinese Medicine

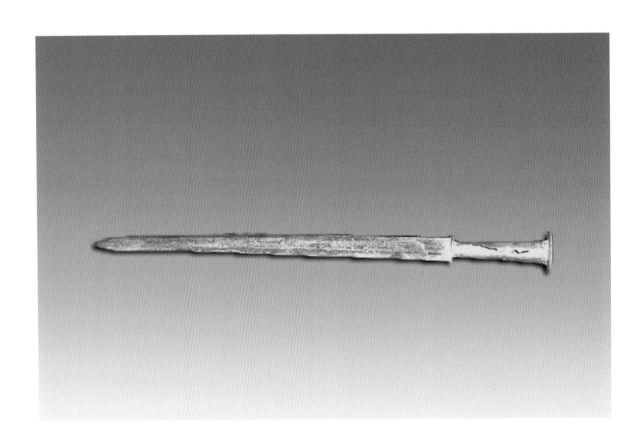

铜剑

战国

铜质

通长 28 厘米，宽 2.8 厘米，重 0.2 千克

Copper Sword

Warring States Period

Copper

Length 28 cm/ Width 2.8 cm/ Weight 0.2 kg

兵器。柳叶形，三棱状，把有一小圆孔。把残。
陕西省西安市征集。

陕西医史博物馆藏

This trigonous sword is a weapon in the shape
of a willow leaf. There is a small round hole on
the hilt which is incomplete. It was collected
from Xi'an, Shaanxi Province.

Preserved in Shaanxi Museum of Medical History

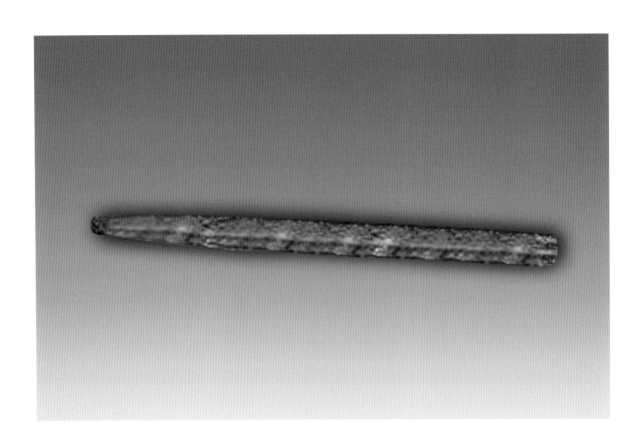

铜扁状器

战国

铜质

长 7.5 厘米，宽 0.4 厘米，重 0.001 千克

Flat Copper Tool

Warring States Period

Copper

Length 7.5 cm/ Width 0.4 cm/ Weight 0.001 kg

长扁状，器身有一凸棱。两头残。生产工具。

陕西医史博物馆藏

The relic is long and flat with a convex ridge on the body. Both ends are damaged. It was used as a tool to work in daily life.

Preserved in Shaanxi Museum of Medical History

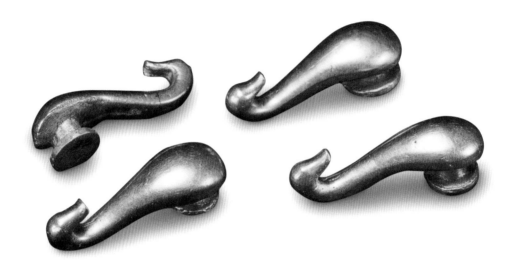

金带钩（4 件）

战国早期

金质

长 4.4 厘米，腹宽 1.4 ~ 1.6 厘米

Golde Belt Hook (Four Pieces)

Early Warring States Period

Gold

Length 4.4 cm/ Belly Diameter 1.4~1.6 cm

钩体作 S 形，下面有柱，素面，工艺精
美，制作考究。具有束住丝带革带的作用。
1978 年湖北省随州市擂鼓墩战国曾侯乙
墓出土。

湖北省博物馆藏

The S-shaped hooks are exquisite and
delicate crafts with studs and no pattern.
They were used for bunching up ribbons or
belts. It was unearthed from Zeng Marquis
Yi Tomb of Leigudun in Suizhou City, Hubei
Province, in 1978.

Preserved in Hubei Provincial Museum

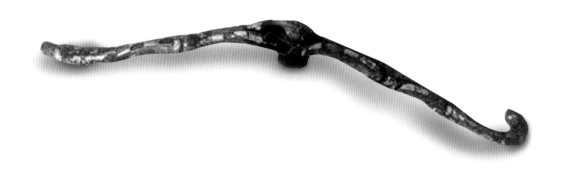

铜带钩

战国

铜质

长 20.5 厘米

Copper Belt Hook

Warring States Period

Copper

Length 20.5 cm

青铜器形质，饰有美丽的花纹。带钩是古代人日常生活的用品，也是衣服上的装饰品。它的作用，除装在革带的顶端用以束腰外，还可以装在腰侧用以佩刀、佩剑、佩印或佩其他装饰物品。

扬州博物馆藏

It is a bronze ware with beautiful patterns. A hook is an daily item for ancient people and an ornament for clothes. It can be mounted on a leather belt to the waist as well as the waist side for sword, seal or other decorative items.

Preserved in Yangzhou Museum

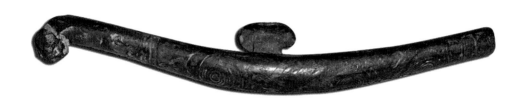

铜衣带钩

战国

铜质

长 13.2 厘米，重 0.1 千克

Copper Belt Hook

Warring States Period

Copper

Length 13.2 cm/ Weight 0.1 kg

弯形，中有一圆纽，一端为钩形。生活器具。

完整无损。陕西省咸阳市秦都区征集。

陕西医史博物馆藏

This curved belt hook has a round knob in the middle and one end of it is hook-shaped. It belongs to life utensil. The intact belt hook was collected by Qindu District of Xianyang City in Shaanxi Province.

Preserved in Shaanxi Museum of Medical History

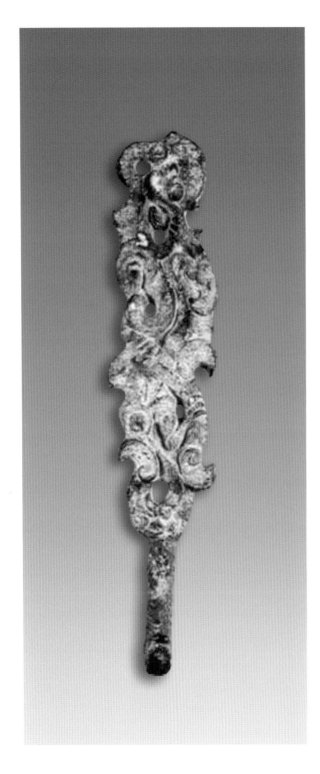

镂雕鹰蛇纹带钩

战国

铜质

长 17.5 厘米

Belt Hook with Hollowed-out Engraved Pattern of Eagles and Snake

Warring States Period

Copper

Length 17.5 cm

钩体扁平微上弧，镂雕双鹰捉蛇图案。蛇
首钩，背面有一圆形钉柱。

山西博物院藏

The belt hook is shaped like a snake head.
The flat body engraved with the design of
two eagles catching a snake bends slightly
upward. On the back is a round stud.
Preserved in Shanxi Museum

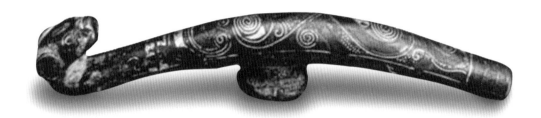

错银云龙纹带钩

战国

铜质

长 10.5 厘米

Belt Hook with Pattern of Cloud and Dragon Smeared with Silver

Warring States Period

Copper

Length 10.5 cm

钩体圆鼓，弧背琵琶形，蛇首钩，背有一圆形钉柱。通体错银饰云龙图案。

山西博物院藏

The belt hook, shaped like a snake head, has a bulging-shaped body, a Pipa-shaped arc back, and a round stud on the back. The whole body is smeared with silver designs of cloud and dragon.

Preserved in Shanxi Museum

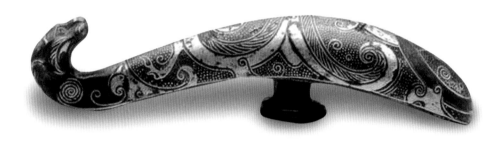

错金银带钩

战国

铜质

长 11.7 厘米，宽 2.3 厘米

Belt Hook with Smeared with Gold and Silver Designs

Warring States Period

Copper

Length 11.7 cm/ Width 2.3 cm

龙首，钩体浑圆，弦背，背部有一圆柱形
钉柱，主体饰涡云纹、弦纹。1973 年陕
西省咸阳市武功县普集乡永台村出土。

咸阳市武功县文管会藏

The hook has a dragon head, round body and
roach back. There is a cylindrical stud on the
back and cloud-like and string patterns on the
body. It was unearthed from Yongtai Village,
Puji Township, Wugong County, Xianyang
City, Shaanxi Province, in 1973.
Preserved in the Cultural Relics Management
Committee of Wugong County, Xianyang City

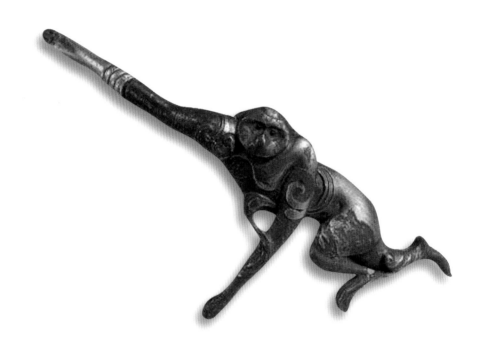

银猿形带钩

战国

银质

通长 16.7 厘米，宽 6.8 厘米

Silver Belt Hook in the Shape of an Ape

Warring States Period

Silver

Length 16.7 cm/ Width 6.8 cm

长臂猿形，振臂，回首，拱身，蹬足，双臂微曲呈钩形，身背有圆形纽。双目镶嵌蓝色料珠，炯炯有神，猿身多处包金，金光灿灿。造型新颖，形象生动，是古代罕见的金银工艺品。1978年曲阜市鲁故城出土。

曲阜市文物局藏

This belt hook is in the shape of an ape with the arms stretching out like hooks, the head looking back, the legs pedaling and the body arching with a round button on its back. The ape's bright eyes are embedded with blue beads. Many parts of its body are overlaid with gold. It is a rare ancient gold-silver handcraft with novel and vivid modeling. This belt hook was unearthed from the city site of Lu States in Qufu in 1978.

Preserved in Qufu Bureau of Cultural Relics

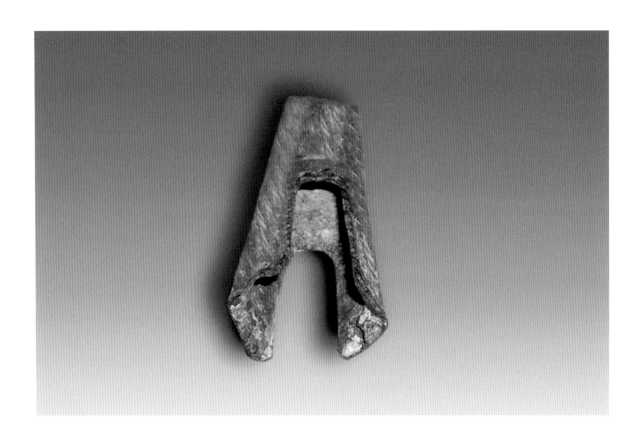

铜铃

战国

铜质

长 5 厘米，重 0.005 千克

Copper Bell

Warring States Period

Copper

Length 5 cm/ Weight 0.005 kg

铃把呈门形，铃呈马鞍形，上有一孔。车饰。
完整无损。内蒙古自治区成陵征集。

陕西医史博物馆藏

This bell, intact and undamaged, is a decoration
for carriage. It has a door-shaped handle. The
bell is in the shape of a saddle with a hole. It
was collected from Mausoleum of Genghis
Khan in Inner Mongolia Autonomous Region.
Preserved in Shaanxi Museum of Medical History

索 引

（馆藏地按拼音字母排序）

Index

参考文献

[1] 李经纬. 中国古代医史图录 [M]. 北京：人民卫生出版社，1992.

[2] 傅维康，李经纬，林昭庚. 中国医学通史：文物图谱卷 [M]. 北京：人民卫生出版社，2000.

[3] 和中浚，吴鸿洲. 中华医学文物图集 [M]. 成都：四川人民出版社，2001.

[4] 上海中医药博物馆. 上海中医药博物馆馆藏珍品 [M]. 上海：上海科学技术出版社，2013.

[5] 西藏自治区博物馆. 西藏博物馆 [M]. 北京：五洲传播出版社，2005.

[6] 崔乐泉. 中国古代体育文物图录：中英文本 [M]. 北京：中华书局，2000.

[7] 张金明，陆雪春. 中国古铜镜鉴赏图录 [M]. 北京：中国民族摄影艺术出版社，2002.

[8] 文物精华编辑委员会. 文物精华 [M]. 北京：文物出版社，1964.

[9] 谭维四. 湖北出土文物精华 [M]. 武汉：湖北教育出版社，2001.

[10] 常州市博物馆. 常州文物精华 [M]. 北京：文物出版社，1998.

[11] 镇江博物馆. 镇江文物精华 [M]. 合肥：黄山书社，1997.

[12] 贵州省文化厅，贵州省博物馆. 贵州文物精华 [M]. 贵阳：贵州人民出版社，2005.

[13] 徐良玉. 扬州馆藏文物精华 [M]. 南京：江苏古籍出版社，2001.

[14] 昭陵博物馆，陕西历史博物馆. 昭陵文物精华 [M]. 西安：陕西人民美术出版社，1991.

[15] 南通博物苑. 南通博物苑文物精华 [M]. 北京：文物出版社，2005.

[16] 邯郸市文物研究所. 邯郸文物精华 [M]. 北京：文物出版社，2005.

[17] 张秀生，刘友恒，聂连顺，等. 中国河北正定文物精华 [M]. 北京：文化艺术出版社，1998.

[18] 陕西省咸阳市文物局. 咸阳文物精华 [M]. 北京：文物出版社，2002.

[19] 安阳市文物管理局. 安阳文物精华 [M]. 北京：文物出版社，2004.

[20] 深圳市博物馆. 深圳市博物馆文物精华 [M]. 北京：文物出版社，1998.

[21] 《中国文物精华》编辑委员会. 中国文物精华（1993）[M]. 北京：文物出版社，1993.

[22] 夏路，刘永生.山西省博物馆馆藏文物精华 [M].太原：山西人民出版社，1999.

[23] 文物精华编辑委员会.文物精华 [M].北京：文物出版社，1957.

[24] 山西博物院，湖北省博物馆.荆楚长歌：九连墩楚墓出土文物精华 [M].太原：山西人民出版社，2011.

[25] 刘广堂，石金鸣，宋建忠.晋国雄风：山西出土两周文物精华 [M].沈阳：万卷出版公司，2009.

[26] 沈君山，王国平，单迎红.滦平博物馆馆藏文物精华 [M].北京：中国文联出版社，2012.

[27] 张家口市博物馆.张家口市博物馆馆藏文物精华 [M].北京：科学出版社，2011.

[28] 浙江省文物考古研究所.浙江考古精华 [M].北京：文物出版社，1999.

[29] 故宫博物院.故宫雕刻珍萃 [M].北京：紫禁城出版社，2004.

[30] 故宫博物院紫禁城出版社.故宫博物院藏宝录 [M].上海：上海文艺出版社，1986.

[31] 首都博物馆.大元三都 [M].北京：科学出版社，2016.

[32] 新疆维吾尔自治区博物馆.新疆出土文物 [M].北京：文物出版社，1975.

[33] 王兴伊，段逸山.新疆出土涉医文书辑校 [M].上海：上海科学技术出版社，2016.

[34] 刘学春.刍议医药卫生文物的概念与分类标准 [J].中华中医药杂志，2016，31（11）:4406-4409.

[35] 上海古籍出版社.中国艺海 [M].上海：上海古籍出版社，1994.

[36] 紫都，岳鑫.一生必知的 200 件国宝 [M].呼和浩特：远方出版社，2005.

[37] 谭维四.湖北出土文物精华 [M].武汉：湖北教育出版社，2001.

[38] 张建青.青海彩陶收藏与鉴赏 [M].北京：中国文史出版社，2007.

[39] 银景琦.仡佬族文物 [M].南宁：广西人民出版社，2014.

[40] 廖果，梁峻，李经纬.东西方医学的反思与前瞻 [M].北京：中医古籍出版社，2002.

[41] 梁峻，张志斌，廖果，等.中华医药文明史集论 [M].北京：中医古籍出版社，2003.

[42] 郑蓉，庄乾竹，刘聪，等.中国医药文化遗产考论 [M].北京：中医古籍出版社，2005.